Anhedonia

and

Affect Deficit States

Anhedonia

and

Affect Deficit States

Edited by
David C. Clark, Ph.D.
and
Jan Fawcett, M.D.
Department of Psychiatry
Rush Medical College
Chicago, Illinois

PMA PUBLISHING CORP.
New York

NOTICE: The editors, contributors, and publisher of this work have made every effort to ensure that the drug dosage schedules and/or procedures are accurate and in accord with the standards accepted at the time of publications. Readers are cautioned, however, to check the product information sheet included in the package of each drug they plan to administer. This is particularly important in regard to new or infrequently used drugs. The publisher is not responsible for any errors of fact or omissions in this book.

Library of Congress Cataloging in Publication Data

Anhedonia and affect deficit states

Papers presented at a symposium held in Chicago in March 1984

Includes index

1. Anhedonia – Congresses. 2. Affective disorders – Congresses. I. Clark, David C., 1949-
II. Fawcett, Jan, 1943- . [DNLM: 1. Affective Disorders – congresses. WM 171 A596 1984]
RC537.A567 1987 616.89 87-2476
ISBN 0-89335-236-5

Printed in the United States of America

About the Editors and Contributors

THE EDITORS

David C. Clark, PhD, is Assistant Professor of Psychiatry and Psychology at Rush Medical College in Chicago.

Jan Fawcett, MD, is Professor and Chairman of Psychiatry at Rush Medical College in Chicago.

THE CONTRIBUTORS

James D. Belluzzi, PhD, is Professor of Pharmacology at the College of Medicine at the University of California at Irvine.

Nancy C. Andreason, MD, PhD, is Professor of Psychiatry at the University of Iowa College of Medicine.

Timothy Collier, PhD, is a postdoctoral research fellow in the Department of Anatomy, University of Rochester School of Medicine and Dentistry.

Martin Harrow, PhD, is Professor of Psychiatry and Behavioral Sciences at the University of Chicago and Michael Reese Hospital.

Donald F. Klein, MD, is Director of Research at the New York State Psychiatric Institute and Professor of Psychiatry, Columbia University College of Physicians and Surgeons.

Henry Krystal, MD, is Professor of Psychiatry at Michigan State University.

Paul E. Meehl, PhD, is Regents Professor of Psychiatry at the University of Minnesota.

Michael F. Pogue-Geile, PhD, is Assistant Professor of Psychology in the Departments of Psychology and Psychiatry at the University of Pittsburgh.

Peter E. Sifneos, MD, is Professor of Psychiatry, Harvard Medical School, and Associate Director of the Psychiatry Service, Beth Israel Hospital.

Larry Stein, PhD, is Professor and Chairman of Pharmacology at the College of Medicine, University of California at Irvine.

Contents

Foreword

DAVID C. CLARK
JAN FAWCETT

In 1897 the French psychologist Ribot introduced the concept of a pathological pleasureless state when he coined the word "anhedonia" ("an insensibility relating to pleasure alone"). Since that time, significant advances in empirical observational research, neuropsychopharmacology, brain neurophysiology, psychoanalysis, and clinical psychology have yielded a mosaic of information about patients and non-patients with anhedonic features. These clues about the etiology and clinical significance of anhedonic phenomena have been difficult to interpret and integrate, however, for several reasons: (a) explicit operational definitions of anhedonia are rarely proposed and applied; (b) dialogue among investigators has often been obstructed by traditional disciplinary boundaries; (c) study design and data interpretation have often been permeated by assumptions about pre-existing relationships between anhedonic states and specific psychiatric disorders (e.g., schizophrenia); and (d) the longitudinal course of anhedonic features in psychiatric patients and non-patients and non-patients has rarely been studied.

Recognizing the need to acquaint investigators and clinicians with the growing body of information about anhedonic phenomena, and the need to facilitate integration and clinical application of this information, we organized a symposium held at The Rush-Presbyterian - St. Luke's Medical Center, Chicago in March 1984, titled: "Anhedonia and Affect Deficit States." The symposium was supported in part by Upjohn, through the good graces of Mr. Joe Bukofsky. The enthusiastic response of the participants, the audience, and many who subsequently requested a record of the proceedings convinced us of the value of organizing the papers presented into a monograph that would be available to biobehavioral investigators and clinicians with a special interest in the area.

The original symposium participants and authors of the papers collected here are distinguished scientists and clinicians engaged in active laboratory and clinical research on fundamental problems related to anhedonia. Donald Klein of Columbia University traces some of his experiences as a clinical psychopharmacologist, and uses them to develop an integrated model of two types of functional pleasure centers operating in the central nervous system. Many will find the figure accompanying his article, illustrating functional structures, feedback loops, pharmacological regulatory mechanisms, and pathology associated with structural or feedback disturbances, to be an heuristic and thought-provoking synthesis of many issues raise throughout the volume. His contribution is a transcript of the original presentation.

Nancy Andreasen of the University of Iowa employs a Kraeplinian approach to objectively operationalize the description of affective blunting through clinical ratings and physical measurements of voice patterns ("acoustic analysis"). Michael Pogue-Geile of The University of Pittsburgh and Martin Harrow of the University of Chicago examine the symptom feature of flat affect in schizophrenic patients as one example of a class of "negative symptoms," and describe the relationship between negative symptoms, positive symptoms, and intellectual dysfunction in the same population. David Clark and Jan Fawcett of Rush-Presbyterian-St. Luke's Medical Center examine the relationship between individual pleasure capacity and depressive state using a patient self-report scale to define pleasure capacity, and summarize the reliability and construct validity of this measure.

Larry Stein and James Belluzzi of the University of California at Irvine examine the phenomenon of positive reinforcement at the cellular level by applying dopamine and cocaine to spontaneously active pyramidal cells in slices of rat hippocampus, and measuring the change in the activity pattern of the neuron that results. Timothy Collier of the University of Rochester reviews the evidence suggesting that opiod neurons participate in the neutral substrates of reward by direct activation of a dopaminergic link in the reward system, rather than subserving an independent opioid reward-related function. In addition, he reports the results of his own study of electrical self-stimulation by rats in a brain location rich in opioid-containing neurons but peripheral to the dopaminergic reward system.

In 1975, Paul Meehl of the University of Minnesota wrote a provocative article reprinted here, postulating that some patients seeking therapy (not neurotic or endogenously depressed) have an inborn feebleness of the physiologic positive reinforcers that normally function as modulators of aversive states. Meehl has written a companion article for the present volume, clarifying and expanding his position in the original paper.

In 1981, Henry Krystal of Michigan State University wrote a stimulating clinical paper reprinted here with substantial modifications discussing the ontogenesis of the hedonic quality of affects, and discussing the interpretation of hedonic and anhedonic phenomena of patients in psychoanalysis. Peter Sifneos of Harvard University discusses the clinical phenomenon of alexithymia, defined as a deficiency in the ability to connect emotions with fantasies, and the anhedonic clinical presentation of many alexithymic patients.

Our aim is to provide a forum where clinicians and investigators studying clinical and laboratory aspects of related phenomena – pleasure and reward systems, flat or blunted affect, joyfulness and joylessness – can compare their operational definitions of anhedonic phenomena, their findings, their interpretations and their integrative models. In this way we hope to create a broader interdisciplinary framework for defining and studying anhedonic phenomena.

Anhedonia
and
Affect Deficit States

1

Depression and Anhedonia

*DONALD F. KLEIN**

The outstanding characteristic of psychiatric patients is that they're very confusing. They present an enormous array of strange attitudes, peculiar emotions and symptoms, overreactions, and underreactions embedded in a complex developmental history. A tangled mess of information is presented and it's all too easy, given this confusing situation, to try to develop some explanatory story or another: "this led to this," "that led to this," "that past experience affected this reaction," etc. Unfortunately, as anybody who has studied the process of psychodynamic formulation knows, any collection of symptoms, signs, and developmental history can be given many equally persuasive dynamic-genetic formulations, and frequently are. So one is left with the question, "What's persuasive about this particular patient?" One usually ends up being persuaded by the theoretical construction one began with.

The nice thing about psychopharmacology is that, when done with proper controls, it is a discrete experimental intervention in a complex system, which is more than can be done most of the time in psychiatry. Therefore one can get some idea of what particular interventions do to a complex reality by tracing out immediate effects, secondary effects, tertiary effects, etc. If done properly, as with double-blind placebo controlled studies, one can assert that a common specific response is actually caused by the pharmacological agent and not by suggestion, psychological impact, rater bias, patient compliance, etc.

I would like to describe my experiences as a clinical psychopharmacologist and use them to develop integrative notions

---

*Supported in part by U.S.P.H.S. Grant MH-30906 – NIMH "New York State Psychiatric Institute, Mental Health Clinical Research Center."

about anhedonia. Pleasure and pleasure regulation are clearly among the important psychological ideas that have been around since the ancient Greeks. Arguments about pleasure and pleasure regulation have formed the center of many of the current psychodynamic theories. Certainly Freud was most interested in pleasure. His particular theory was primarily one of excitation reduction, and implied that there is only one sort of pleasure. These ideas were given more centrality by Sandor Rado in his discussions of hedonic regulation, but the basic drive reduction framework was preserved.

My first work on a psychiatric ward was in a state hospital, back in the early 1950s. We didn't have antidepressants or antipsychotics; essentially all we had was ECT. Our patients were often severely depressed people who weren't eating and paid little attention to their surroundings. Their sleep was markedly disturbed, they were frequently suicidal, and were in awful shape. ECT was the only useful treatment and indeed helped many in a most remarkable way.

I was casting around at the time to see if there were alternative interventions. The only one that made any sense was dextroamphetamine. I tried giving such depressed patients amphetamine in substantial doses. Occasionally and unpredictably, patients would exhibit a sudden but transient improvement of mood. For a number of other patients, amphetamine seemed to convert their illness from a retarded depression to an agitated depression; that wasn't much of a gain. That indicated to me that whatever amphetamine was doing, its effects were quite peripheral to the pathophysiological defects associated with the kinds of depression that required hospitalization and often responded to ECT.

My next illuminating psychiatric experience was two years spent running the admission and withdrawal unit at the U.S.P.H.S. Narcotics Hospital in Lexington, Kentucky. I knew nothing about drug addiction, so the work was extremely informative. One of the things that interested me was that the addicts had distinct tastes with regard to what it was that turned them on. Some preferred cocaine and some liked morphine. Some liked them simultaneously mixed together as a "speedball" and affirmed that it was quite different from either morphine or cocaine alone.

This led me to question the existence of a single functional pleasure response. Both cocaine and morphine, taken intravenously, produce a tremendous rush of pleasure, but the addict had no trouble at all distinguishing between the drugs and expressing a preference for one over the other. Further, the behavior associated with taking either morphine or cocaine is quite different. Cocaine doesn't satiate. When the patient takes cocaine, he goes on a run. He'll take a snort, get high, take another snort, get higher, take another snort, get higher, until he runs out of cocaine. The cocaine addict calls that "going on a run." Amphetamine addicts (speed freaks) do exactly the same thing. They go on and on until they run out.

That's not true of opiate addicts. Opiate addicts take a shot and then "go on the nod." They become quiet, sedated, sleepy, and quite indifferent to things around them. Emotionally, they are "cool," which means imperturbable. The cocaine addict, however, is not indifferent at all; he's flying, but often very focused. He's not paying attention to everything going on around, but rather pays absorbed attention to one narrow thing. So you have the peculiar situation where the cocaine run is a positive feedback loop that does not manifest satiation, whereas morphine self-administration produces quick (although temporary) satiation.

There are certain similarities between these drug effects and aspects of our normally occurring pleasurable activities. Certain activities generate positive feedback loops. These activities are primarily in the foraging, hunting, searching and socializing area. A very good example of a pleasurable activity that often produces a crescendo of massive joyful excitation is sexual foreplay. This is a good example of pleasure in an excitatory situation and seems to contradict the belief that all pleasure derives from excitation reduction.

On the other hand, there are activities such as having a big meal or sexual orgasm which result in pleasure, satiation and a quiet sedation. These activities appear to function as a negative feedback loop and turn themselves off. The analogy between positive-feedback and negative-feedback pleasures, on one hand, and the different effects of cocaine and morphine is interesting but unlikely to be as simple as it first appears.

At Hillside Hospital in 1959, we studied imipramine. It was an antidepressant, we were told. We didn't know what an antidepressant was, but figured it must be a super-amphetamine, something like cocaine. The first thing that happened to our severely retarded depressed patients on imipramine was that they slept better, then their appetite improved and some weeks later their mood normalized. Whatever this drug was, it did not act like a stimulant. It was a horse of a different color.

It became obvious that not all depressives got better on tricyclics, so we tried to figure out who got better on tricyclics and who didn't. Some severe patients were interested in nothing, enjoyed nothing, and their mood could not be improved by positive rewards. They sat quietly in the corner, unresponsive, or were pacing around the ward agitated, wringing their hands and appealing for help. They were either in a retarded or an agitated depression.

Those terribly ill patients were precisely the ones who had a terrific normalizing response to imipramine. Further, their case histories usually showed illness of a phasic sort. They were often quite ordinary people, living a quite ordinary life, when they abruptly went into a depressive phase, sometimes after a precipitant and sometimes not.

There was another group of people who also complained of feeling terribly depressed, and asserted "Nothing interests me, I'm bored, apathetic, I can't get anything out of life, it's terrible." Then on the wards you would find them animatedly chatting and complaining if there were not enough amusements. The first depressed group that I talked about (retarded or agitated) didn't want amusements since amusements did them no good. Further, they couldn't anticipate any good.

The second group by and large did not respond to tricyclic antidepressants. We did not use MAO inhibitors then because they were considered dangerous drugs, but since that time we have developed substantial interest in and respect for them.

A third group we saw at Hillside were people who were enormously involving of the staff. They were histrionic, seductive, unstable people. The staff regularly divided themselves up into those who said that "This poor soul requires saving and I'm going to do it," and those who said, "She's a terrible, malingering hysteric and let's get rid of her." This was before the time the term "borderline" became so popular, but nowadays I'm sure they would be called borderline.

The outstanding affective complaints of patients in the third group were also of an intense lack of interest, boredom and emptiness. Strangely enough, they tended to overeat and oversleep, whereas the kind of depressive who responded to tricyclics usually had anorexia and insomnia. Patients in the third group also did not benefit from tricyclic therapy. If anything, tricyclics seemed to make them worse.

There were other clinical observations that must be integrated into a theory relating hedonic process and psychopathology. We randomly assigned severe depressives to either placebo, impramine or chlorpromazine (which is usually not considered an antidepressant, but an antipsychotic). Nonetheless, we found that chlorpromazine worked as well as impramine. It wasn't just reducing their agitation. Their mood got better at about the same time as mood improved in the patients on tricyclics. That was not a fluke. There have been several other studies demonstrating that antipsychotics are effective mood-alleviating agents for severe depression (Felger, 1965; Hollister et al., 1966, 1967; Klein, 1967; Overall et al., 1966; Paykel et al., 1968; Raskin et al., 1970). That's really in complete contradiction to current catecholaminergic theories.

Also, some depressed patients treated with tricyclics exhibited about a 70% response. You could describe them as sleeping alright, having a restored appetite, going home on pass, and having sexual relations, but still just not as interested in activities as they ought to be. Further, they resist having to go back to work. They feel they can't swing it, and are not quite healthy enough to go back to work. At that point, adding a small dose of amphetamine to the tricyclic would suddenly increase their interest and energy, and they would return to work. Note that at the beginning of treatment, giving these patients amphetamines would have done them no lasting good.

It sounds as if these patients went through a two-step process in recovering from their illness. The first step was the restoration of what one might refer to as "consummatory pleasures": pleasures in biological drive reduction such as pleasure in sexual orgasm, eating, and perhaps sleep. The second step was restoration of the pleasure associated with pursuit: being able to go after things with interest. The continued deficiency of pursuit pleasures seemed responsive to amphetamine, once the consummatory pleasures had been normalized.

Once I drew this distinction between consummatory pleasures and appetitive (pursuit or foraging) pleasures, I could make better sense of the patients who said they felt terribly depressed, but who were socializing, and chatting it up on the ward. These patients never had inhibition of their consummatory pleasures. While they said they were very depressed, they still enjoyed sex and food; they simply weren't going after it. If it was given to them on a silver platter they could enjoy it, but the pursuit factor was gone. They were apathetic. Further, their apathetic mood was to some degree non-autonomous. If somebody came along, jollied them up, and said they were terrific and admirable and attractive and wasn't it wonderful how they were bravely withstanding the tremendous trouble they were going through – that would lighten their mood. For a short period of time they would feel OK, but then would slump right back into an apathetic mood when the input stopped. They were often referred to as character disorders.

The term *character disorder* is an attempt to explain chronic maladaptation. Affective disorders have traditionally been conceptualized as periodic or phasic states – they come and they go. But it is possible there are such things as chronic affective disorders that are often attributed to some rigid attitudinal or defensive structure, which we call character, rather than to an affective difficulty.

How can you tell? One way is by making a pharmacological intervention. If an individual's chronic difficulties in managing his life respond to a mood-improving pharmacological intervention, that's substantive evidence that the difficulty is not characterological (i.e., habitual) because it's hard to conceive of a drug changing a person's character. Not impossible, but unlikely. Patients who have non-autonomous depressions with preservation of consummatory pleasures but inhibition of appetitive (foraging, searching, hunting) pleasures, tend to exhibit a chronic history. They often said they had trouble since they were a teenager. A question we routinely ask is "Have you had six good continuous months since you've been a teenager? Six months in a row when things were fine?" Most of our patients say "no" to that one. That's chronic.

I hypothesize that there are two functional pleasure systems, and that a defect in the consummatory system is always accompanied by a defect in the appetitive pleasure system. The terms appetitive and consummatory may seem complicated. One analogy is the difference between pleasures of the hunt and pleasures of the feast. They're not the same thing. If one has inhibition of the ability to experience the pleasure of the feast, the pleasures of the hunt are also inhibited. Further, I hypothesize that a defect in the consummatory pleasure system always produces an autonomous depression. That is, you can't jolly a person with a consummatory defect into a pleasant mood.

I postulate that tricyclics work directly on pathological consummatory inhibition and only secondarily influence appetitive inhibitions. For those depressed patients who still retain their appetitive inhibitions, giving amphetamine improved matters and they were able to pursue pleasure. But as long as their consummatory system was inhibited, they could not respond to the amphetamine.

On the other hand, the MAO inhibitors seemed to work directly on the appetitive system, so that the person with an atypical non-autonomous depression, who maintained consummatory but not appetitive pleasures, was helped by MAO inhibitors rather than by the tricyclics. Fred Quitkin, Mike Liebowitz, other colleagues and I have since done a randomized trial to tricyclics, MAO inhibitors, and placebo. We've studied about one hundred and twenty atypically depressed patients so far, and our results are quite clear. The MAO inhibitors worked better than the tricyclics for appetitive system depressions. The tricyclics, I was surprised to find, worked better than placebo. So the MAO inhibitors are much more effective than placebo and also more effective than tricyclics. The tricyclics do have some activity; so that's something to figure out.

Since tricyclics work well on primary consummatory inhibition but not so well at primary appetitive inhibition, would it follow that, conversely, MAO inhibitors (which work well at appetitive inhibition) should not work as well on consummatory inhibition? In fact, there's one big study of the two hundred and fifty largely endogenous inpatients done by the British Medical Research Council in which they compare MAO inhibitors with placebo; the MAOIs had no beneficial effect whatsoever (Klein, Gittelman et al., 1980). Our group at Columbia decided to check that out ourselves. We recruited two series of twelve endogenous outpatients and gave them phenelzine or tranylcypromine in open trials. They weren't severely ill, but they had a distinct lack of both consummatory and appetitive pleasures. Such patients in previous placebo control trials had about a 20% response rate. On the MAOIs we observed a response rate of 75%. We will do a placebo controlled study to be sure, but I think the MAOI benefit is really there.

There is a hint that the patients who didn't get better on MAO inhibitors were the most severe of the endogenous patients. There may be something there. Probably there is heterogeneity among endogenomorphic depressives. One subgroup suffers from a primary consummatory inhibition and the tricyclics may be necessary for that group. That is the group whom I think of as being most phasic, most abrupt in onset, and least chronic.

There may be another group where the appetitive inhibition spreads and develops a secondary consummatory inhibition. There is a parallel clinical pattern. We have seen a number of patients who have "atypical" depression. They have phases where they overeat, oversleep and have a reactive mood. Then at some point, things go sour and their illness converts into an endogenomorphic depression. They can't sleep and they lose their appetite.

So this is not a clear enduring categorical distinction whereby patients never change categories. There also seems to be the possibility of a severity transition, so that people who begin with an apparently pure appetitive inhibition can progress to develop both

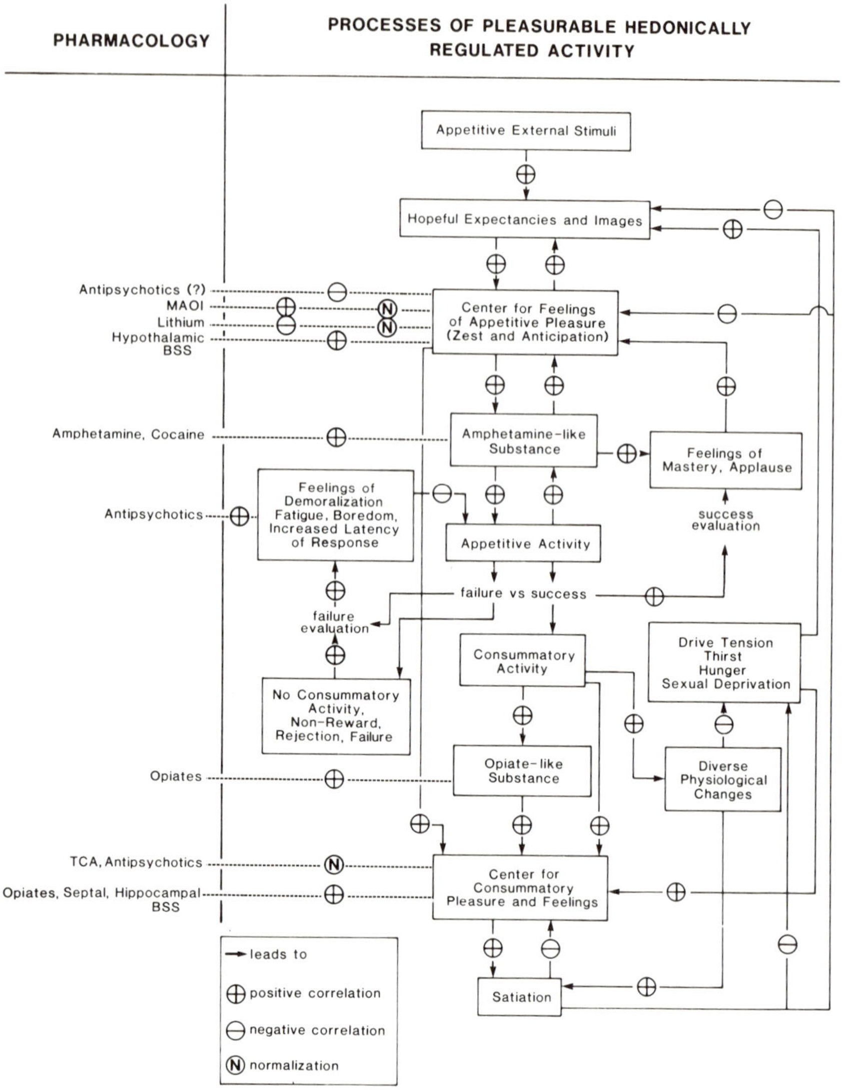

Figure 1.1. Process of pleasurable hedonically regulated activity.

appetitive and consummatory inhibitions. Therefore, among people who have consummatory inhibitions, we postulate both primary and secondary consummatory inhibitions. If that were true, and MAO inhibitor benefit was limited to relieving primary appetitive inhibition, we should be able to predict who among the endogenous

PATHOLOGY
Appetitive Pleasure Deficit Chronic Decreases in Chronic Schizophrenia
Phasic Decreased Appetitive Pleasure a) Demoralization b) Atypical Depression Increased Appetitive Pleasure a) Mania b) Hypomania
Phasic Decreased Amphetamine-like Substance (ALS) a) Bulimia b) Narcolepsy c) Kleine - Levin
Chronic Decrease ALS a) Atypical Depression #2 b) Fatigue, Neurasthenia c) Akinesia d) Secondary Amphetamine Addiction
Decreased Opiate-released Substances → Secondary Opiate Addiction (???)
Phasic Decreased Consummatory Pleasures → Endogenomorphic Depression
Increased Consummatory Pleasure a) Unio-Mystica (?) b) Ecstasy
Decreased Satiation → Bulimia (?) Increased Satiation → Anorexia Nervosa (?)

patients are going to respond to MAO inhibitors and who should not. We haven't done that yet.

The monoamine oxidase inhibitors actually affect at least two brain systems: monoamine oxidase A and monoamine oxidase B. Monoamine oxidase A is the one that regulates norepinephrine, serotonin and tyramine. Monoamine oxidase B regulates phenylethylamine. Phenylethylamine is a substance that differs from amphetamine by only one methyl group. It is the prime substrate for MAO B.

If you believe that appetitive inhibition indicates that an amphetamine-like substance was either not being created or not being as effective as it should be, then you could guess that a pure MAO B inhibitor would be particularly effective in that group of patients. Now there is a pure MAO B inhibitor called deprenyl. We've done a substantial open trial on atypical depressives which indicated that deprenyl works. John Mann has done a controlled study that indicates it works for atypical depressives (Mann, Francis et al., 1982). There has been one study in England on endogenous depressives which reports it doesn't work (Mendis, Pare et al., 1981), which would be fine, but there is still another Belgian study (Mendlewicz and Youdim, 1983) which says it does work for endogenous depressives. So that's yet another pharmacological tool which may help us to figure out these complex issues. Is there some way to integrate this confusing melange of clinical and pharmacological observations? There is, I think, but the model is somewhat more complex than the New York City subway system.

There are two types of pleasure; appetitive pleasure and consummatory pleasure. Appetitive pleasure guides and incites people into activities that will eventually result in consummatory pleasures. The consummatory pleasures then result in a phase of satiation with relative inactivity.

Figure 1.1 illustrates some hypothesized relationships between these two functional pleasure centers and other psychological and neurotransmitter systems. In the figure, pluses refer to positive correlations. If two components are connected by a plus, they move up and down together in step. Minuses refer to negative correlations. If one node goes up, the other node is likely to go down and vice versa. "N" refers to "normalization," wherein a deranged reactivity is brought back to normal.

At the top of the figure I suggest that the organism may be presented with appetitive external stimuli, hinting at opportunities for eventual consummatory action. Hopeful expectancies and images are generated when one is confronted with appetitive stimuli. Further, there is a positive feedback loop associated with the appetitive drive state. That is, if you're in a state of heightened drive it generates hopeful expectancies and fantasies. These hopeful expectancies then stimulate the center for feelings of appetitive pleasure. In other words, it makes you feel good when you are contemplating the possibility of consummatory pleasure, as any daydreamer can tell you. The appetitive center makes you feel good about both the anticipation and pursuit of consummatory pleasure.

Clark and Fawcett have developed what they call a pleasure scale (Fawcett, Clark et al., 1983). Are they measuring pleasures at the appetitive or consummatory level? I suggest they're measuring pleasures at the appetitive level, because they are really asking the person to imagine how they're going to feel.

I hypothesize the center for feelings of appetitive pleasures releases an amphetamine-like substance (ALS), and that there's a positive feedback loop because the amphetamine-like substance in turn stimulates the center for appetitive pleasure. This substance may be phenylethylamine or perhaps some cocaine-like agent. The identity of the stimulating agent is obscure.

The amphetamine-like substance also stimulates appetitive activity: hunting and pursuit activity. The pleasures that people get in sports, running, jogging and all sorts of active play are appetitive pleasures. A great deal of sports activity can easily be understood as mock hunting activity. The hunger-suppressing effects of amphetamine also fit this model since you don't want to be distracted by hunger contractions while chasing a rabbit.

I also suggest that everyone has a central comparator that evaluates the success of appetitive activities. If that evaluator indicates that things are going well, you are getting applause, you are getting close to your goal object, your goal object is giving you signals that things are fine, so then you have a positive feedback loop with a crescendo of good feeling, activity, expansiveness and goal approach.

Conversely, if you're in a failing situation, your pursuit activity is not working. This gets evaluated, inhibits your appetitive pleasure center, and is associated with feelings of demoralization, fatigue, boredom, and hopelessness. These then result in a decrease in appetitive activity, which serves an appropriate conservative function, if you are in a non-rewarding environmental patch.

Various pharmacological agents and pathological states can be understood at the appetitive level, considered as a positive feedback loop. The pathological state that I think is clearest is when the center for appetitive pleasure just isn't working. Then I think you end up with an atypical depression, apathy, disinterest, but usually (at least initially) maintain consummatory pleasures.

What happens if the positive feedback loop works too well? The brakes on the positive feedback system no longer work. That, I think, is probably manifest as mania. The manic person is extraordinarily energetic, expansive, searching, hunting, and everything looks terrific to him. Everything is going to work well, he's going to go and do it and it's going to be wonderful.

It's also conceivable you might have abrupt decreases in the amphetamine-like substance associated with appetitive regulation, which pulls the rug out from under, in a phasic way. This may produce syndromes such as narcolepsy, Kleine-Levin syndrome and bulimia. Bulimia is a good example, since amphetamines have a hunger inhibiting character. The bulimic patient binges as if suddenly disinhibited from a voracious carbohydrate hunger. Interestingly, bulimics have been satisfactorily treated with both amphetamines and MAO inhibitors (but also tricyclics).

Do anti-psychotics decrease appetitive pleasure? People on anti-psychotics seem somewhat apathetic. You can argue whether that's an aspect of Parkinsonian akinesia or an actual decrease in appetitive pleasure. The MAO inhibitors seem to normalize or actually stimulate the center for appetitive pleasure. Lithium seems to normalize or actually inhibit responsivity to some degree in some people. Certain sorts of brain self-stimulation (BSS), as in hypothalamic brain self-stimulation, also result in a non-satiating crescendo of activity that may relate to this center's activity. Amphetamine and cocaine may substitute for or release the amphetamine-like substance.

Let us move on to the consummatory phase of the hunt. The consummatory activities in particular are eating, drinking, sexual orgasm and perhaps sleeping. These activities incur diverse physiological changes: blood glucose goes up, cholecystokinin releases, etc. However, consummatory pleasures may have in common the release of some sort of opiate-like substance or substance that opiates release. That opiate-like substance could be enkephalin or endorphin, or something along those lines, which stimulates the center that produces feelings of consummatory pleasure. That is not a positive feedback loop. The opiate-like substance triggers a consummatory pleasure center discharge, which then fires off the satiation center. The satiation center sends up a negative message to both the appetitive and consummatory centers saying, "Enough already; you've done your job; relax for a while."

What would be pathology at the level of the consummatory center? A decrease in the responsivity of the consummatory pleasure center would result in something that strongly resembles an endogenomorphic depression.

Is there anything that looks like a consummatory or satiating excess besides I.V. opiates? We can speculate. Some psychotic individuals have intense, participatory states in which they are at one with the universe or in a state of desireless Nirvana. These experiences sound a good deal like the reports of heroin addicts, mystics, and some epileptics. Also, interference with the satiation mechanism might relate to such illnesses as anorexia nervosa and bulimia. The anorexic will tell you, "I ate one cookie and that's enough; I'm really full; I don't want anymore." Whereas the bulimic says, "I'm empty inside; no matter what I put in, I just can't get enough. I just have this big hollow feeling." Clearly these ideas are not even close to being proven. Nonetheless they may stimulate some hypothesis testing and eventually demonstrate some practical value for psychopharmacological practice.

REFERENCES

Fawcett, J., Clark, D.C., Scheftner, W.A., and Gibbons, R.D. (1983). Assessing anhedonia in psychiatric patients: The Pleasure Scale. *Arch. Gen. Psychiatry*, 40:79-84.

Felger, H.L. (1965). Depressed hospitalized psychotic patients treated with chlorprothixene concentrate. *J. New Drugs*, 5:242-248.

Hollister, L.E., Overall, J.E., Shelton, J., Pennington, V., Kimbell, I., and Johnson, M. (1967). Amitriptyline, perphenazine and an amitriptyline-perphenazine combination in different depressive syndromes. *Arch. Gen. Psychiatry*, 17:486-493.

Hollister, L.E., Overall, J.E., Johnson, M.H., Shelton, J., Kimbell, I. and Brunse, A. (1966). Amitriptyline alone and combined with perphenazine in newly admitted depressed patients. *J. Nerv. Ment. Dis.*, 142:460-469.

Klein, D.F. (1967). Importance of psychiatric diagnosis in prediction of clinical drug effects. *Arch. Gen. Psychiatry*, 16:118-126.

Klein, D.F., Gittelman, R., Quitkin, F. and Rifkin, A. (1980). *Diagnosis and Drug Treatment of Psychiatric Disorders: Adults and Children* (Second edition). Baltimore: Williams & Wilkins.

Mann, J.J., Francis, A., Kaplan, R.D. et al. (1982). The relative efficacy of l-deprenyl, a selective monoamine type B inhibitor in endogenous and nonendogenous depression. *J. Clin. Psychopharm.*, 2:54-57.

McGrath, P.J., Quitkin, F., Harrison, W., and Stewart, J.W. (1984). Treatment of melancholia with tranylcypromine. *Am. J. Psychiatry*, 141:288-289.

McGrath, P.J., Quitkin, F., Harrison, W. and Stewart, J.W. (Unpublished data). Treatment of melancholia with phenelzine.

Mendis, N., Pare, C.M.B., Sandler, M., Glover, V. and Stern, G.M. (1981). Is the failure of (-) deprenyl, a selective monoamine oxidase B inhibitor, to alleviate depression related to freedom from the cheese effect? *Psychopharmacology*, 73:87-90.

Mendlewicz, J. and Youdim, M.B.H. (1983). L-deprenil, a selective monoamine oxidase type B inhibitor, in the treatment of depression: A double blind evaluation. *Brit. J. Psychiatry*, 142:508-511.

Overall, J.E., Hollister, L.E., Johnson, M. and Pennington, V. (1966). Nosology of depression and differential response to drugs. *J.A.M.A.*, 195:946-948.

Paykel, E.S., Price, J.S., Gillian, R.U., Palmer, G., and Chesser, E.S. (1968). A comparative trial of imipramine and chlorpromazine in depressed patients. *Brit. J. Psychiatry*, 114:1281-1287.

Raskin, A., Schulterbrandt, J.G., Reatig, N., and McKion, J. (1970). Differential response to chlorpromazine, imipramine and placebo; A study of subgroups of hospitalized depressed patients. *Arch. Gen. Psychiatry*, 23:164-173.

2
Affective Flattening: Evaluation and Diagnostic Significance

NANCY ANDREASEN

> . . . We meet everywhere the characteristic fundamental features of the Freudian trend of investigation, the representation of arbitrary assumptions and conjectures as assured facts, which are used without hesitation for the building up of always new castles in the air ever towering higher, and the tendency to generalization beyond measure from single observations. I must frankly confess that with the best will I am not able to follow the trains of thought of this "metapsychiatry," which like a complex sucks up the sober method of clinical observation. As I am accustomed to walk on a sure foundation of direct experience, my Philistine conscience of natural science stumbles at every step on objections, considerations and doubts, over which the lightly soaring power of imagination of Freud's disciples carries on without difficulty. (Emile Kraepelin, 1919)

The tension between the need for careful empirical observation and the need to soar above facts and to generalize is always great. The above remarks of Emile Kraepelin, directed primarily at his arch-rival Eugen Bleuler (whom Kraepelin considered to be a follower of Freud), illustrate the tension. In particular, Kraepelin is objecting to Bleuler's notions that the symptoms of schizophrenia can be understood as evolving from psychodynamic "complexes," many of which are fundamentally sexual. While Bleuler searched the horizons to find underlying theoretical causes, Kraepelin planted his feet squarely in the clinic and was content to simply describe what he saw in his patients. While Bleuler craved generalities, Kraepelin relished particularities.

In the midst of a collection of papers devoted primarily to enlarging our theoretical understanding of affective deficits and anhedonia, this paper will take a more Kraepelinian approach. It will describe attempts to operationalize objectively the description of affective blunting either through clinical ratings or physical measurements. This approach is based on the belief that we must be able to quantify and measure emotional and mental phenomena if we are also to be able to understand them. To paraphase William James, general theories concerning affective deficits and anhedonia in mental illness must be forged "in the teeth of irreducible and stubborn facts" (Whitehead, 1925).

My own approach to understanding affective deficits is thus a "bottom-up" rather than a "top-down" one. I would propose that our understanding of affective flattening, as well as other phenomena that occur in mental illness, should be built through an orderly and sequenced program that attacks the problem in step-wise fashion:

> *Stage One:* Clinical description, involving the development of reliable clinical ratings of the manifestations of affective flattening.
>
> *Stage Two:* Physiological description, involving the development of techniques for measuring the physical manifestations of affective flattening.
>
> *Stage Three:* Examination of mechanisms and causes, involving the development of techniques for understanding the symptom in terms of brain structure and function.

CLINICAL DESCRIPTION

The first detailed clinical description of affective flattening appears in the work of Kraepelin (1919) who described it as follows:

> The singular indifference of the patients toward their former emotional relations, the extinction of affection for relatives and friends, of satisfaction in their work and vocation, in recreation and pleasures, is not seldom the first and most striking symptom of the onset of disease.

> The patients have no real joy in life, "no human feelings" . . . . Hopes and wishes, cares and anxieties are silent; the patient accepts without emotion dismissal from his post, being brought to the institution, sinking to the life of a vagrant, the management of his own affairs being taken from him . . . He lives one day at a time in a state of apathy. The background of his disposition is either a meaningless hilarity or a morose and shy irritability.

In addition to the above manifestations, Kraepelin also notes that patients may show emotional inappropriateness, loss of moral sentiments as manifested by antisocial behavior, loss of sympathy as manifested by indifference and want of understanding for the misfortunes of others, disappearance of delicacy of feeling as manifested by inappropriate sexual behavior or excretory behavior, and a decrease in sensitivity to bodily discomfort as manifested by diminished sensitivity to pain.

Bleuler also considered affective flattening an important clinical symptom. As is well known, he thought it to be one of the fundamental symptoms of schizophrenia, which he believed to be pathognomonic of the disorder, as distinguished from accessory symptoms, which might occur in other illnesses. He describes affective flattening (1950) as follows:

> "Emotional deterioration" stands in the forefront of the clinical picture. It has been known since the early years of modern psychiatry that an "acute curable" psychosis became "chronic" when the affects began to disappear. Many schizophrenics in the later years cease to show any affect for years and even decades at a time. They sit about the institution to which they are confined with expressionless faces, hunched-up, the image of indifference . . . . even in the less severe forms of the illness, indifference seems to be the external sign of their state: an indifference to everything – to friends and relations, to vocation or enjoyment, to duties for rights, to good fortune or bad.

Anyone who works with patients suffering from major mental illnesses cannot help but agree with Kraepelin and Bleuler concerning the clinical importance of this symptom. Not only does it occur frequently, but, as Bleuler suggests, it may be an important marker for chronicity and poor prognosis. Yet researchers interested in nosology and phenomenology have been reluctant to incorporate it into standarized diagnostic systems used for research because of a concern that it may have poor reliability. Standard research criteria such as the Washington University Criteria (Feighner and colleagues, 1972) or the Research Diagnostic Criteria (Spitzer, Endicott and Robins, 1977) do not make any references to affective flattening, while it is given only very minor emphasis in DSM-III.

More recently, however, several attempts have been made to make ratings of affective flattening more reliable. Abrams and Taylor recently reported a scale that may be used with good reliability to evaluate blunted affect, and at about the same time I reported a similar scale developed independently of their work (1978).

My scale, "The Affect Rating Scale," was developed by trying to identify behavioral indices of affective flattening (Andreasen, 1979). Unlike some symptoms of mental illness, such as delusions or dysphoria, the evaluation of affect does not depend on the patient's self-report or description of his thoughts and feelings. Rather, affect is rated by observing the patient's emotional responsiveness. I selected the items on my scale by asking myself what aspects of a patient's behavior a skilled clinician notices when he or she attemps to evaluate affective flattening. After giving the matter some thought, I developed a list of nine phenomena, all of which are behavioral. In general, clinicians usually decide that a patient fails to look them in the eye, does not smile back when smiled at, and lacks other physical indices of emotional responsivity. The nine items on the scale are as follows:

1. *Unchanging facial expression:* The facies appears wooden, mechanical, and frozen and does not change expression or changes less than normally expected, as the emotional content of discourse changes.
2. *Decreased spontaneous movements* The patient or subject sits quietly throughout the interview and shows few or no spontaneous movements; he or she does not shift position, move legs, move hands, etc., or does so less than normally expected.
3. *Paucity of expressive gestures:* The patient does not use his body as an aid in expressing his ideas through such means as hand gestures, sitting for-ward in his chair when intent on a subject, leaning back when relaxed, etc. This may occur in addition to decreased spontaneous movements.

4. *Poor eye contact:* The patient avoids looking at the interviewer or using his or her eyes as an aid in expression. He or she appears to be staring into space even when talking.
5. *Affective nonresponsivity:* The patient fails to smile or laugh when prompted. This may be tested by smiling or joking in a way that would usually elicit a smile from a normal individual. The examiner may also ask, "Have you forgotten how to smile?" when smiling himself.
6. *Inappropriate affect:* Affect expressed is inappro-priate or incongruous, not simply flat or blunted. Most typically, this manifestation of affective disturbance takes the form of smiling or assuming a silly facial expression when talking about a serious or sad subject. (Occasionally patients may smile or laugh when talking about a serious subject that they find uncomfortable or embarrassing; although their smiling would seem inappropriate, it is due to anxiety and therefore should not be rated as inap-propriate affect.)
7. *Lack of vocal inflections:* While speaking, the patient fails to show normal vocal emphasis patterns. Speech has a monotonic quality, and important words are not emphasized through changes in pitch or volume. The patient may also fail to change volume with changes of subject, so that he does not drop his voice when discussing private topics or raise it as he discusses things that are exciting or for which louder speech may be appropriate.
8. *Slowed speech*: Speech seems slowed, with longer pauses between words, phrases, or clauses than seems normal.
9. *Increased latency of response:* The patient takes a longer time to reply to questions than is usually considered normal.

A four-point rating scale was written for each of these definitions. For example, the scale for "unchanging facial expression" is as follows:

1 = not at all (patient is normal or labile).
2 = mild (some decrease in facial expressiveness).
3 = moderate (facial expressiveness is significantly decreased).

4 = severe (no change in facial expression throughout the interview.

In addition, an item was written for making a global rating of affective flattening, which uses a similar four-point scale.

These definitions were then used to rate a total of 69 patients drawn from Iowa Psychiatric Hospital, Mount Pleasant, and the Iowa City Veterans' Hospital. These patients met Research Diagnostic Criteria for mania (N = 19), depression (N = 20), and schizophrenia (N = 30), with the additional proviso that the patients with schizophrenia had been ill for at least six months. Although patients were usually evaluated within the first week after admission, nearly all were receiving medication such as lithium, phenothiazines, or tricyclics. Since phenothiazines often produce symptoms suggestive of affective flattening, it should be noted that nearly all of the patients with schizophrenia (95 percent) were receiving neuroleptics, as were many of those with mania (55 percent) and some of those with depression (33 percent).

After informed consent was obtained, the patients were interviewed by a pair of raters (one of whom acted as an observer) who were blind as to the patient's diagnosis and who used a standard 45-minute structured interview that covered a wide range of both neutral and affect-laden topics, such as religious or political beliefs, interests and hobbies, or descriptions of family members. The patient's symptomatology was not discussed in order to minimize diagnostic clues. One of the raters was an experienced psychiatrist (NCA); the other two were clinical research scientists with master's level training in psychology and several years of clinical and research experience.

Table 2.1 indicates the interrater reliability, as shown by intraclass correlation coefficient, for the nine components of affective flattening and the global rating. Seven out of ten ratings have an intraclass correlation coefficient greater than .5, usually considered as an acceptable minimum for adequate interrater reliability. The three variables with poor reliability tended to occur rather infrequently, making reliability difficult to assess and probably spuriously low. These results suggest that an empirical approach to affective flattening may produce adequate reliability.

Table 2.1 also shows the frequency of the various components of affective flattening in the three diagnostic groups; the number and percentage of patients receiving a rating of mild or greater is used as an indicator of frequency. In spite of the fact that many patients with mania were receiving phenothiazines, relatively few received ratings

Table 2.1
Frequency of Affective Flatteining in Manics

	Intra-class R	MANICS (N = 19)		DEPRESSIVES (N = 20)		SCHIZOPHRENICS (N = 30)	
		N	%	N	%	N	%
1. Unchanging facial expression	.7361	2	10.5	8	40.0	16	53.3
2. Decreased spontaneous movements	.7103	4	21.1	10	50.0	11	36.7
3. Paucity of expressive gestures	.5775	7	36.8	11	55.0	17	56.7
4. Poor eye contact	.7977	3	15.8	7	35.0	11	36.7
5. Affective non-responsitivity	.3697	0	0	1	5.0	9	30.0
6. Inappropriate affect	.2904	0	0	1	5.0	6	20.0
7. Lack of vocal inflections	.5133	4	21.1	12	60.0	16	53.3
8. Slowed speech	.6775	1	5.3	6	30.0	5	16.7
9. Increased latency of response	.0708	1	6.3	2	10.0	3	10.0
10. Global rating of affective flattening	.6330	4	21.1	11	55.0	19	63.3

of 2 or greater on any of the variables. On the other hand, both depressive patients and schizophrenic patients tended to have relatively high ratings on many variables, particularly unchanging facial expression, decreased spontaneous movements, paucity of expressive gestures, and the global rating.

These data suggest that when an empirical and observational approach is taken to define affective flattening, good reliability can be achieved. All items on the scale that have a relatively high base rate tend to have an interrater reliability that ranges from acceptable to excellent.

These data also suggest that affective flattening is not pathognomonic of schizophrenia nor omnipresent in it. Affective flattening is also common in depression and cannot be used to discriminate between schizophrenia and the depressive pole of affective disorder. (In an analysis of variance, the F-ratio for the global rating was 6.05, $p < .025$, with the patients with depression and schizophrenia differing significantly from those with mania.)

The issue of the relationship between phenothiazines and affective flattening is also an important one. Nearly all manic and schizophrenic patients in this study were on neuroleptics; consequently, the increase in affective flattening in the schizophrenic patients cannot be attributed primarily to the effects of neuroleptics. On the other hand, it may seem surprising that any patients with mania received positive ratings for affective flattening. This result is probably a mixture of the effect of neuroleptics and the fact that severe manics may manifest "stuporous mania." Ideally, it would be desirable to do similar ratings in drug-free patients.

PHYSIOLOGICAL CORRELATES

While improvement in our ability to evaluate affect clinically is a necessary first step in operationalizing our concepts about it, it is also useful to attempt to develop some quantitative physical measurement of affective flattening. Many possibilites are available, such as autonomic response to painful or aversive stimuli, or indices of reactivity measured while the patient watches an emotionally-charged videotape. Indeed, measurements of this sort seem an imperative next step in order to improve our understanding of the concept of affect and its diagnostic significance.

One objective physical measurement of affective flattening employed in our work has involved characteristics of voice patterns, otherwise known as "acoustic analysis" (Andreasen, Alpert and Martz, 1981). Since the 1950s, a number of investigators have explored the relationship between emotional states and such vocal characteristics as fundamental frequency (pitch) and amplitude (loudness) (Roessler and Lester, 1967; Alpert et al., 1963, 1967, 1977; Hargreaves et al., 1965; Ostwald, 1964; Simonov and Frolow, 1973;

Williams and Stevens, 1969, 1972; Mahl, 1964; Starkweather, 1964; Huttar, 1968). These studies have used the technique of converting speech to a visual analog that may then be studied independently of content. The use of computerized averaging has permitted the study of relatively large samples and has reduced the signal:noise ratio. These previous studies suggest that measuring vocal characteristics using such techniques may be a worthwhile objective tool for evaluating emotional states such as anger, fear, and depression.

We therefore hypothesized that vocal characteristics could provide a useful measure of affective flattening. This hypothesis was based on the clinical recognition that patients with flatness of affect often speak in a monotonic manner. Acoustically, this monotonic quality should be reflected by a decrease in the variability of both amplitude and frequency. Our preliminary work in this area suggests that acoustic analysis may indeed be a good objective measure of affective flattening.

In this study, we examined a subset of the patients described above for whom measurements had been collected using the Affect Rating Scale. They included 15 patients with major depressive disorder, 19 patients with manic disorder, and 27 patients with schizophrenia. For the purposes of this study, the global rating was used to classify the patients into the following two groups: flat and non-flat. Patients were classified as flat if they had a global rating or 2 or greater. On this basis, 31 patients were considered to have flatness of affect and 30 to be non-flat.

The voice analysis was done on tape-recorded samples of the 45-minute structured interview described above. Microphone distance was standardized at 6 inches from the patient's mouth. Volume levels were set for each patient so that the loudest speech was at maximum volume unit (VU) level. The interviews were then completely transcribed, and areas inappropriate for acoustic analysis (e.g., because of a loud background noise) were noted on the transcript. Since patients varied in the length of their response to specified interview questions, it was not possible to select a single standard topic for voice analysis in the middle of the interview.

The acoustic measures that we studied appear in Figure 2.1.

A run (or utterance) is defined as a signal above a predefined threshold without a silence of more than 0.3 seconds. A pause is defined as a period below threshold greater than 0.3 seconds. Within each run, there are individual peaks that correspond to syllables. In our analysis, the duration to each peak is noted and the log of its height is taken as the peak amplitude. We also record the funda-

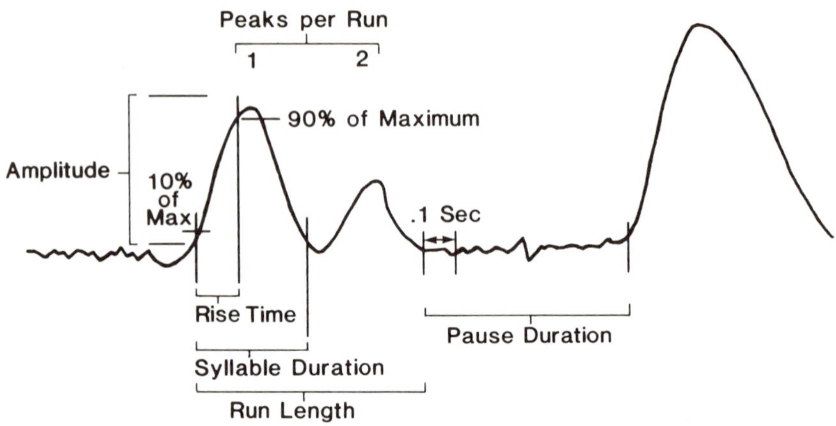

Figure 2.1. Measures of features of acoustical waveform of human speech. Not shown: frequency. This is a fundamental frequency, or basic pitch, of the voice.

mental frequency for each peak. The time from the beginning of a syllable to its peak is the "rise time" and is measured as a percent of the total syllable duration. We also measured the length of each peak, which corresponds to syllable duration. Thus the means and standard deviations for the following seven variables were available for investigation: amplitude, or loudness; frequency, or pitch; syllable duration; rise time; run length; peaks per run; and pause duration. These variables were checked repeatedly for each patient and were found to have excellent reliability when samples from the same occasion were compared.

Computerized averaging was used to calculate the means and standard deviations for each of these variables for each patient. For a variety of reasons, the standard deviations or variances were thought to be of more importance than the means. First, flatness of affect, if reflected in monotonic speech, would be measured by decreases in variability more powerfully than by decreases in specific variables such as amplitude or frequency. Second, our method for recording and sampling requires further refinement in order to make some of the mean measurements meaningful. For example, both amplitude and frequency are affected by the sex of the patient, and the flat and non-flat groups did not have equal sex ratios. Further, amplitude may be affected by head movement.

We have divided our variables into two groups: measures of dynamics and intonation, and measures of rate. Our hypotheses concerning these variables are shown in Table 2.2. Because patients

Table 2.2
Hypotheses Concerning Flatness

Variable	Flatness
Dynamics and Intonation	
Amplitude	—
S Amplitude	↓
Frequency	—
S Frequency	↓
Rise time	—
S Rise time	—
Rate Measures	
Syllable duration	-
S Syllable duration	↓
Run length	↓
S Run length	↓
Peaks per run	—
S Peaks per run	—
Pause length	↑
S Pause length	—

with flat affect are likely to have monotonic speech, we would expect them to have a significantly lower variation in both amplitude (S-amplitude) and frequency (S-frequency). Further, since flat patients also speak with a somewhat staccato quality, they should have a decrease in the variability of their syllable duration. Further, since they tend to have "poverty of speech," this should be reflected in decreased run length, decreased variance of run length, and increased pause length.

The results of our analyses are shown in Tables 2.3 and 2.4.

Table 2.3
Dynamics and Intonation in Affective Flattening

	Not Flat (N = 30)		Flat (N = 31)		
Variable	$\bar{x}$	SD	$\bar{x}$	SD	p
Amplitude	6424.94	734.67	6331.59	761.13	NS
S-Amplitude	784.56	116.45	708.01	132.02	.002
Frequency	444.16	58.44	422.17	43.64	NS
S-Frequency	35.38	12.57	29.05	9.70	.031
Rise Time	2115.12	482.55	1882.34	433.77	.034
S-Rise Time	1322.12	276.12	1191.82	269.25	NS

Data concerning dynamics and intonation are given in Table 2.3. As hypothesized, the flat group tended to have significantly less variability in both amplitude and frequency as measured by S-amplitude and S-frequency. The flat group also tended to speak with a lower frequency (which probably reflects a greater number of males in this group) and to have a smaller rise time. Although the difference in frequency is probably not meaningful, the difference in rise time may be. The rise time is a measure of the amount of time it takes a speaker to reach peak amplitude when he is speaking each word. The smaller the mean rise time, the more staccato the speech is likely to sound. Since the speech of patients with affective flattening often has a staccato quality in addition to its monotonic quality, this result is not surprising.

Rate measures for the two groups are given in Table 2.4. There are no significant differences in the means or variances of syllable duration, as was hypothesized. On the other hand, the flat group has a shorter run length, less variance in run length, fewer peaks per run, less variance in peaks per run, and longer pause length. Thus, the flat group tended to speak briefly, to say fewer words in a run, and to pause longer before resuming speech again. These measures perhaps reflect a related cognitive aspect of affective flattening, poverty of speech, since they probably reflect a diminution in amount, flow, and spontaneity of speech.

Table 2.4
Rate Measures of Affective Flattening

Variable	Not Flat (N = 30) $\bar{x}$	Not Flat (N = 30) SD	Flat (N = 31) $\bar{x}$	Flat (N = 31) SD	p
Syllable duration	224.94	24.36	227.66	22.41	NS
S-Syllable-duration	90.53	11.94	92.30	12.60	NS
Run length	169.11	56.63	143.48	37.91	0.510
S-run-length	139.10	59.53	132.57	35.69	0.160
Peaks per run	61.69	20.22	53.49	12.99	0.050
S-peaks-per-run	50.75	21.62	49.82	12.52	0.057
Pause length	113.16	45.39	134.15	59.45	0.055
S-Pause-length	107.86	14.89	140.67	122.20	NS

This work suggests that voice analysis may provide a useful objective measure of affective flattening. The patients who displayed flatness of affect showed vocal characteristics that are consistent with their lack of emotional spontaneity and responsiveness. That is, they tended to speak in a monotonic and staccato manner, as shown by decreased variation in the loudness and frequency of their speech and by a decrease in rise time. We have now collected a second sample and are attempting to determine whether or not we can replicate our original findings. In addition, we are exploring additional techniques for developing objective physical measurements of affective flattening.

ANATOMIC LOCALIZATION

Affect is the outward and visible sign of internal neuronal behavior. However, neuroscientists are only beginning their efforts to map cognition and emotion in the brain. Thus, for the moment we can only speculate, using very insufficient data, as to the anatomical localization of a symptom such as affective flattening.

One region that might be implicated is of course the prefrontal or frontal system. Animal studies have shown that prefrontal lesions generally result in impoverishment of emotional life and social isolation (Fuster, 1980). Experience with prefrontal leucotomy in human beings has shown that these patients also have profound abnormalities in affect and emotion (Fuster, 1980). These patients tend to be indifferent to themselves, to others, and to their surroundings. They are also indifferent about the future and seem to be unable to modulate their affect in response to either actual change or anticipated change in their environment. In addition, patients with frontal lesions show the indifference to social mores and the diminution in social sensibilities that Kraepelin described so vividly as manifestations of affective flattening in schizophrenia. Finally, the frontal system has been implicated in recent PET scan and regional blood flow work in schizophrenic patients (Ariel et al., 1983; Mathew et al., 1981; Ingvar and Franzen, 1974; Buchsbaum et al., 1982).

A second brain region that may represent an important source of affect is the limbic system. Animal research has indicated that there are several portions of the limbic system involved in such important components of affect as ability to feel pleasure or pain, to seek self-stimulation, and to seek rewards. Both the hypothalamus and the septal region have been found to play a part in emotional behavior in animals (Isaacson, 1982). Patients who have received frontal leucotomy have of course in a sense had limbic lesions, since the severed tracts have often included the cingulate gyrus, a frontal region that is also part of the limbic system. It should also be noted that Stevens (1982) has reported rather consistent findings of hypothalamic and periventricular pathology in patients suffering from schizophrenia, and she has noted some correlation between these findings and affective flattening observed prior to death.

A final, and somewhat less obvious, portion of the brain that must be considered is the basal ganglia. This region may provide a motor component for affective flattening, if not a psychological or emotional component. Patients with Parkinson's disease often have an appearance of affective flattening, as revealed in their mask-like facies and akinesis. They do not usually, however, have a subjective sense of emotional blunting, although they may experience the painful affect of depression. Thus our experience with Parkinsonian patients suggests that we should perhaps think of affect in terms of both a motor or expressive part and an emotional or receptive part. In any intact person these two parts would interact with one another, just as the expressive and receptive language regions interact with one another. In the case of Parkinsonian patients, we may be observing a person who has a pure expressive deficit in affect without a receptive deficit. This observation is interesting because it implies that the localization of affect, when it is finally mapped, is likely to be highly complex.

REFERENCES

Abrams, R., Taylor, M.A. (1978). A rating scale for emotional blunting. *American Journal of Psychiatry*, 135:226-229.

Alpert, M., Anderson, L.T. (1977). Imagery mediation of vocal emphasis in flat affect. *Archives of General Psychiatry*, 34:208-212.

Alpert, M., Frosch, W.A., Fisher, S.H. (1967). Teaching the perception of expressive aspects of vocal communication. *American Journal of Psychiatry*, 124:106-115.

Alpert, M., Kurtzberg, R.L., Friedhoff, A.H. (1963). Transient voice changes associated with emotional stimuli. *Archives of General Psychiatry*, 8:362-365.

Andreasen, N.C. (1979). *The Affect Rating Scale.* Available from the author on request.

Andreasen, N.C. (1979). Affective flattening and the criteria for schizophrenia. *American Journal of Psychiatry*, 136:944-947.

Andreasen, N.C., Alpert, M., Martz, M.J. (1981). Acoustic analysis: An objective measure of affective flattening. *Archives of General Psychiatry*, 38:281-285.

Ariel, R.N., Golden, C.J., Berg, R.A., et al. (1983). Regional cerebral blood flow in schizophrenics. *Archives of General Psychiatry*, 40:258-263.

Bleuler, E. (1950). *Dementia Praecox or the Group of Schizophrenias*, translated by J. Zinkin. New York: International Universities Press, Inc.

Buchsbaum, M.S., Ingvar, D.H., Kessler, R., et al. (1982). Cerebral glucography with positron tomography. *Archives of General Psychiatry*, 39:251-259.

Diagnostic and Statistical Manual of Mental Disorders, 3rd edition (1980). Washington, D.C.: American Psychiatric Association.

Feighner, J.P., Robins, E., Guze, S.B., et al. (1972). Diagnostic criteria for use in psychiatric research. *Archives of General Psychiatry*, 26:57-63.

Fuster, Joaquin (1980). *The Prefrontal Cortex: Anatomy, Physiology, and Neuropsycho logy of the Frontal Lobe*. New York: Raven Press.

Hargreaves, W.A., Starkweather, J.A., Blacker, K.H. (1965). Voice quality in depression. *Journal of Abnormal Psychology*, 70:218-220.

Huttar, G.L. (1968). Relations between prosodic variables and emotions in normal American English utterances. *Journal of Speech and Hearing Research*, 11:481-487.

Ingvar, D.H., Franzen, G. (1974). Abnormalities of cerebral blood flow distribution in patients with chronic schizophrenia. *Acta Psychiatrica Scandinavica*, 50:425-462.

Isaacson, R. L. (1982). *The Limbic System*, 2nd edition, New York: Plenum Press.

Kraepelin, E. (1919). *Dementia Praecox and Paraphrenia*, translated by R.M. Barkley. Edinburgh: E & S. Livingstone.

Mahl, G.F. (1964). Some observations about research on vocal behavior. In Rioch, D., Weinstein, E. (Eds.), *Disorders of Communication*, Volume 42. Research Publications of the Association for Research in Nervous and Mental Disease. Baltimore: Williams & Wilkins, pp. 466-483.

Mathew, R.J., Meyer, J.S., Francis, B.J., et al. (1981). Regional cerebral blood flow in schizophrenia: A preliminary report. *American Journal of Psychiatry*, 138:112-113.

Ostwald, P.F. (1964). Acoustic manifestation of emotional disturbance. In Rioch, D., Weinstein, E. (Eds.), *Disorders of Communication,* Volume 42. Research Publications of the Association for Research in Nervous and Mental Disease. Baltimore: Williams & Wilkins Company, pp. 450-465.

Roessler, R., Lester, J.W. (1976). Voice predicts affect during psychotherapy. *Journal of Nervous and Mental Disease*, 163:166-176.

Simonov, P.V., Frolow, M.V. (1973). Utilization of human voice for estimation of man's emotional stress and state of attention. *Aerospace Medicine*, 44:256-258.

Spitzer, R.L., Endicott, J., Robins, E. (1977). *Research Diagnostic Criteria for a Selected Group of Functional Disorders*, 3rd edition, New York: New York State Psychiatric Institute, Biometrics Research.

Starkweather, J.A. (1964). Variations in vocal behavior. In Rioch, D., Weinstein, E. (Eds.), *Disorders of Communication*, Volume 42. Research Publications of the Association for Research in Nervouc and Mental Disease. Baltimore: Williams & Wilkins, pp. 424- 449.

Stevens, J.R. (1982). Neuropathology of schizophrenia. *Archives of General Psychiatry*, 39:1131-1139.

Quoted by Alfred North Whitehead (1925). *Science and the Modern World.* New York: The Macmillan Company, Chapter 1.

Williams, C.E., Stevens, K.N. (1972). Emotions and speech: Some acoustical correlates. *Journal of the Acoustical Society of America*, 52:1238-1250.

Williams, C.E., Stevens, K.N. (1969). On determining the emotional state of pilots during flight: An exploratory study, *Aerospace Medicine*, 40:1369-1372.

3

Hedonic Capacity: Some Conjectures

PAUL E. MEEHL

One important historical consequence of the discoveries of Freud and his co-workers has been the widespread acceptance among psychotherapists (of various persuasions, many of whom would not describe themselves as "Freudian") of what might be labeled the impedance view of almost all psychological aberration. In suggesting this locution I do not mean to pseudo-solve theoretical or therapeutic problems by a piece of novel semantics. Because I want to avoid discussing theoretical and technical differences among psychotherapists who would object to formulations in the "proper Freudian" terminology (e.g., resistance, defense, superego anxiety) while I focus attention upon a view that is ubiquitous and rarely questioned, I use the term impedance for it is descriptive and fairly neutral with respect to other theoretical and tactical controversies.

The essence of the impedance view of psychological malfunctioning and suffering can be simply stated: Most (all?) persons who seek professional help because of what they (or their friends, relatives, or internists) perceive as "psychological problems" are in psychological trouble because of the existence of certain mental forces or structures that impede effective behavior and resultant subjective impulse gratification. From this simple principle – that the trouble with neurotics is some psychological force impeding their functioning – it should be obvious that the theoretical posture and the therapeutic

---

Reprinted with permission from the *Bulletin of the Menninger Clinic*, 39:295-307, copyright 1975, The Menninger Foundation.

technique should be primarily focused on removing those impeding forces. Thus, the classical view of the essence of therapy* rests basically upon this impedance conception of psychological distress and social or medical malfunction.

Of course, there are other broadly uncovering or insight-oriented psychotherapies (e.g., the Rogerian) that cannot be formulated in Freudian terms. These psychotherapies, despite their avoidance of such concepts as resistance, working through, or interpretation, share with the classical Freudian position the basic notion that people suffer psychologically, malfunction socially, or produce psychosomatically-mediated symptoms primarily because certain psychological counterforces do exist and operate as impedances to pleasure-seeking, gratification, loving, working, problem-solving, effective social conduct, and the like.

It is not my purpose in this paper to refute the impedance doctrine, which I happen to believe has a great deal of truth to it despite the difficulty in making a rigorous scientific case for it to our skeptical academic brethren.†

This brief article is avowedly conjectural in nature. Since I am a neo-Popperian in my philosophy of science, I am unabashedly presenting a conjecture (in Popper's sense) without having any substantial so-called "foundations" or "confirmation" in support of it (Popper 1959, 1962, 1972; Bunge 1964; Schilpp 1974). I think the conjecture is interesting and worth pursuing, and if the reader asks - despite my neo-Popperian philosophic orientation - where I "get such ideas from," I would say they come primarily from a mixture of casual observation with some thirty years experience as a psychotherapist. I do not, let me hasten to add, view the latter as very strongly evidentiary, since it appears obvious from the contemporary therapeutic scene that sane, intelligent, bedoctored persons of good will can spend thousands of hours listening to patients or clients and emerge with radically different views as to just "what is wrong with them." But being a good neo-Popperian, I do not believe that a conjecture requires positive support. All you need to justify in propounding a conjecture is the existence of a problem; and, so far as I

---

* I use the phrase "essence of therapy" to refer to interpretations whose technical function is to enable the patient's ego to tolerate less distorted derivatives, characterized over the long run as a process of working through his resistances - equating resistance with defense as it occurs in the therapeutic situation.

† See Meehl, 1970.

know, the existence of psychological problems is not in dispute! So while I will mention some scattered bits and pieces of evidence, partly clinical, partly experimental, and partly psychometric that seem to me to bear upon this conjecture of mine, I want to emphasize the highly speculative nature of this contribution. Its aim is modest, being to call attention of clinicians and theoreticians to an interesting and important possibility which is researchable in principle and which, at the very least, we can stack up against our own clinical experience in trying to help people with their psychological difficulties.

My conjecture, like the tradition of the impedance doctrine, can be stated (as a first approximation) quite simply: In the impedance doctrine, we assume that all neurotics are suffering an impairment of both their positive gratifications and effective instrumental behaviors. Such impairment is a result of the impeding influence of negative affects (notably the anxiety signal) and the defensive systems acquired to handle them. This formula constitutes a theoretically biased orientation on our part. What we know of the mental machinery (whether from the laboratory or from common observation) should lead us to suspect that there is, in many people, an equally important quantitative influence in the opposite direction, namely, a quantitative feebleness or weakness of the positive reinforcers that normally function as "softeners" of aversive states (such as rage and fear). Such persons - who might be characterized as being at the low end of the continuum for basic hedonic capacity - are not, therefore, suffering from impedances; and a psychotherapy oriented fundamentally toward clearing away impedances may be inappropriate for them.

Before the discovery of specific positive and negative reinforcement centers in the central nervous system, such a theoretical conjecture had not only considerable armchair plausibility but also corroboration by anecdotal and clinical observation. Anybody who observes children is struck by the remarkable range of individual differences in what appears to be their capability for experiencing pleasure, even at an early age.* The impedance theory implies that the enjoyment potential of the apparent low hedonic type is impaired by interference from defensive characterological rigidities, excesses of the anxiety signal, and the like. I am, of course, aware that this answer would be the standard one to my conjecture. However, my aim is to call that standard answer into question by raising the possibility

* See Escalona, 1968.

that just as there are some organisms whose pleasures are impeded by fear, so are there other organisms whose fears are insufficiently softened, attenuated, or, I may even say, impeded by adequate pleasure. Still, at the anecdotal level, people totally unlearned in technical psychodynamics are well aware that if you want, for instance, to discuss an emotionally-charged topic with a potential enemy, among the things you are well advised to do is feed him and sex him and otherwise make him feel good, with the purpose of generating an overall psychological state that will be more or less incompatible with anxiety and rage. But, there is also the old "Wild West" maxim: "Some men are just born three drinks behind."

In the course of intensive psychotherapy, many patients – by no means always depressed or schizoid in makeup – spontaneously report (and more could do so if the therapist were alert to the idea of basic hedonic deficiency) that even as children they noticed they were different from the others because they had the distinct impression that everything seemed to be more fun for other children than for themselves. Here again one who is strongly committed to the impedance interpretation of neurosis can usually succeed in eliciting information supporting the view that the child was being impeded from adequate pleasure by some aversive state, such as social fear. But I think it takes some forcing of the facts to make all of the cases fit this pattern, even phenomenologically. My clinical impression is that some persons, whether reporting childhood or current adult situations, do not provide us with adequate support for the postulation of an impeding anxiety signal or characterological rigidity of a defensive nature; they seem simply not to get the usual quantitative "kick" out of life's purported positive experiences.

Speaking now as an academic psychologist, taking off my clinician's hat for the moment, I suggest this conclusion could have been theoretically expected. In practically any physical or psychological trait we have bothered to investigate systematically there are tremendous differences. Given our direct experimental knowledge of the existence of Olds (+) centers in the brain, I think most psychologists would be willing to guess, with relatively high armchair confidence, that considerable differences among persons exist – and I include here "normal" persons not seeking psychotherapeutic help – in the distribution, number, density, or reactivity of these positive reinforcement ("pleasurable") brain centers. Secondly, the growing mass of data in behavioral genetics suggests that almost any temperamental disposition in which there exists important individual differences – especially one known from direct laboratory research to reside in specific neuroanatomical loci – is, at least to some degree, inheritable.* Since we take for granted today that not everybody is born with an equal innate disposition to the anxiety signal, we should also take for granted that one important source of the differences between those who fall ill of a neurosis and those who, despite life's stresses and frustrations, manage to stay reasonably healthy lies in differential susceptibility to anxiety. Therefore, I conjecture, clinicians and theoreticians ought to consider seriously the possibility that not only are some persons born with more cerebral "joy-juice" than others but also that this variable is fraught with clinical consequences.

It should be apparent from what I have said that I do not always think of what Rado called "anhedonia" as a pathological entity. My conjecture involves the usual academic psychologist's emphasis upon a normal individual differences variable; however, this emphasis considerably alters the likelihood that social or medical pathology will arise at the statistical extremes of the distribution. Since I suppose very few people come to a psychotherapist for help because life is too much fun, our clinical sampling of the two ends of this distribution is biased. But I am convinced that "high-joy" people do exist; and I should be surprised if my readers, in contemplating their range of acquaintances, disagree with me. There are persons who seem able to take considerable pleasure from almost any circumstance not distinctly loaded with aversive components and for whom the most ordinary experiences appear to be a source of considerable gratification. I conjecture that these people are the lucky ones at the high end of the hedonic capacity continuum, i.e., they were "born three drinks" ahead.

Because activation of the Olds (+) centers has a tendency to inhibit, soften, or attenuate the negative (aversive) experiences with which everyday life, alas, so often abounds, this normal range of individual differences has the potential for becoming extremely important clinically. I suggest that a person who has the misfortune of being on the low end of the hereditary hedonic capacity continuum – a fact not, in itself, clinically pathological in my view – may experience life as unduly burdensome and stressful for the simple reason that although he has to put up with the same kinds of annoyances, anxieties, and threats the rest of us do, his difficulties are not being softened or statistically counterbalanced by adequate hedonic "kicks."† In fact,

* See Meehl, 1974-75 for references to genetic factors.

† This notion runs counter to the impedance theory but has an analogous quantitative meaning.

some patients have spontaeneously reported something very close to this assessment. Most psychotherapists I know have had patients (again, I emphasize, patients who are not severely depressed or convincingly schizotypal) who say such things as, "Well, you know, I have to get up in the morning when I hear the alarm clock ring and go out and shovel the walk and all that kind of junk, and what do I really get out of it? I mean, it strikes me that life is often pretty much a big pain in the neck - it just isn't worth it; it's more trouble than it's worth. And I really don't understand why most of my friends seem to feel differently about it." Sometimes such a statement is a typical impedance neurosis complaint. Sometimes it is a cry for help. Sometimes it is part of what my colleague Schofield (1964) would describe as the "philosophical neurosis." But sometimes – and, I suggest, more commonly than most clinicians are ready to recognize – it is a substantially accurate account of the patient's reinforcement schedule (Ferster & Skinner 1957), mainly attributable to his inheriting unlucky polygenes that put him at the low end of the hedonic capacity continuum. So, in effect, he is complaining to the therapist that he is like a white rat in a Skinner box who spends most of his time pressing the level to keep the shock turned off but does not receive very many pellets – and, for him, unfortunately, this simile represents the literal truth.

I should like to digress slightly to discuss my views on depression since they relate to the present conjecture about hedonic capacity. I believe (partly on the basis of clinical impressions) that there are at least five, and possibly as many as seven, distinguishable kinds of depression (not associated with coarse brain disease or other organic illness). Since it is not appropriate to document this claim here, I will simply list the types: (1) endogenous bipolar (manic-depressive), (2) endogenous unipolar, (3) retroflex rage, (4) object loss, (5) extinction depression (the only kind Skinner recognizes and the kind greatly underestimated by psychotherapists in the psychodynamic tradition), (6) depression secondary to schizotypy, and (7) depression secondary to low hedonic capacity. Skinner's extinction depression applies to a person who becomes depressed not because of any complex intrapsychic dynamics and not because an inherited psychotic depression gene is activated, but because he has recently been put on a quantitatively unsatisfactory reinforcement schedule, perhaps quite by happenstance. For instance, if I hit a period during which I do not sell much insurance and my wife does not have orgasms and my friends do not laugh at my jokes and my new car is full of "bugs," I will tend to become depressed.* The layman often understands this kind of depression more readily than the psychotherapist. "No wonder the poor guy is depressed. Everything bad has happened to him all at once lately."

My conjecture about depression secondary to low hedonic capacity is a kind of physiological equivalent to Skiller's extinction depression. However, instead of the external social Skinner box administering an inadequate number of positive reinforcers, those "objective" pellets that are being delivered are not psychophysiologically received as reinforcers because of the aberrated hedonic parameter. Of course, the important practical difference is that extinction depression will either go away by itself (if it is merely a random "bad run" of extinction trials) or can be altered by helping the patient into a different social Skinner box in which the pellet deliveries will happen more frequently, e.g., change jobs, wives, cars or whatever. Although with this kind of patient a therapist may be operating mistakenly upon a pure impedance view of neurosis, he nevertheless may do the patient a great deal of good. In the course of interpreting the alleged impedances there can occur a cognitive restructuring and a freeing up of risk- taking trail and error; and, as a result, the patient moves into a positive reinforcement schedule and undergoes significant quantitative improvement. However, for the patient whose depression is secondary to his being genetically located at the low end of the hedonic capacity continuum, no such effective behavior is available. Although Rado (1956) has talked about teaching patients (mainly schizotypes) to learn to live with a "scarcity economy of pleasure," I must confess I have not found his writings on this problem very practical.

I must emphasize that, given the conjectural nature of this brief contribution, I make no pretense whatever to a systematic literature search of either experimental or differential psychology studies. Instead, I shall mention certain well-known, exemplifying studies that are, at least consistent with the proffered conjectures. The classic undergraduate textbook example of interfering with a conditioned anxiety signal by associating the anxiety elicitor with a positive (reinforcing) stimulus is Jones' (1924) report on how a child's conditioned fear of a rabbit was overcome by contiguous feeding. Then

* See Meehl, 1962b.

we have Farber's (1948) finding that the well-known rigidity or "response fixation" under anxiety in the T-maze (using rats as subjects) could be reduced by feeding in the experimental situation, although no reinforcement contingencies were involved. "Counter-conditioning" or "reciprocal inhibition" experiments provide the theoretical basis underlying Wolpe's therapeutic method (Wolpe & Lazarus 1966). Brady and Conrad's (1960) study revealed that direct intracrannial limbic system self-stimulation of positive centers could markedly attenuate a conditioned aversive emotional response in rats and monkeys, although not in cats.* I would also consider relevant the analgesic effect of masturbation reported by Marchand (1961) and, along similar lines, the regrettable and (according to my colleagues in psychopharmacology) rather consistent correlation between the potency and the dependability of anti-pain drugs and their addictive and euphoria-inducing properties. In the search for better pain relievers, repeated claims have been made that some new drug (e.g., Demerol) is just as effective as morphine but less addictive. Such claims have regularly proven incorrect.† The psychological element in subjective physical pain is universally recognized today and hardly in need of further documentation. How much something hurts, even though it has a clear-cut peripheral origin in organic disease, depends considerably (some pain experts would argue for the word mainly) upon what might be broadly called the anxiety component involved.

At present it would not be possible to marshal a comparable body of clinical or research evidence from either differential psychology or behavior genetics. As for differential psychology, I will mention, as a plausible candidate for identification with hedonic capacity, Cattell's (1935) surgency, an individual differences factor which he says shows up consistently not only in his work but also in the work of most investigators but usually under other names (Cattell, 1957). For example, English and English (1958) define it as "a trait inferred to account for behaviors that are cheerful, lively, responsive, social, trustful." In a statistical study of personality ratings on patients by psychotherapists (Meehl et al. 1971), my colleagues and I were surprised (since neither we nor the rating clinicians were routine users of Cattell's factor scheme) to detect a

---

* See also Olds, 1958; Hernandez-Peon, 1964, especially the mutual antagonism diagram 17 on p. 199; Wilson & Davison 1971, replied to by Reid, 1973.

† See, for example, Modell, 1961.

large individual differences factor which we tentatively called surgency and which Cattell* unreservedly agreed with on reading the item content. Readers of that paper (Meehl et al., 1971) might reasonably argue that our surgency factor is too much permeated with social or interpersonal item content to qualify as a hedonic potential variable, and I would want to give that argument due weight. However, while I cannot present a rebuttal here, I suggest that in a variety of clinical and research contexts – not only those involving hedonic capacity – one might expect an overrepresentation of social content in differential psychology studies (1) because of the relatively higher clinical visibility of the social indicators of psychological factors to raters, and, in my view more significantly, (2) because parametric differences in basic temperamental variables reflected in acquired molar behavior traits should theoretically be activated by an intermittent reinforcement schedule as is the case for social dispositions. My hunch is that this factor explains why the aversive drift invariably seen in schizotypes tends – although there are striking individual exceptions – to be largely reflected in the interpersonal area (Meehl 1962a, 1964, 1972b). The reinforcement schedule the external world imposes upon most of us with regard to most domains of instrumental behavior (such as the act of reaching for a pencil or, as we see in many schizotypes, seeking aesthetic and intellectual pleasures) tends, at least in the statistical sense, to be more "consistent"† than is true of most interpersonal responses.

Finally, as to the inheritability of hedonic capacity, I must repeat that I rely here (probably much more than most of my readers would consider legitimate) on an armchair formula: Any basic temperamental variable that shows pronounced individual differences, especially one for which specific neuro-anatomic loci are known, will to some considerable extent be variable because of genetic differences.‡ As it happens, Lieblich and Olds (1971) have reported successful genetic selection for readiness to respond to intracranial stimulation as a positive reinforcer.

Admittedly these miscellaneous clinical, psychometric, and experimental findings provide only weak corroboration for my

* Personal communication.

† In Skinnerian language, one might describe them as having a smaller VR environmental parameter.

‡ See, for example, Williams, 1956, Meehl, 1972a and the research literature cited therein.

composite conjecture. Strong tests are imaginable, but probably must await better assessment technologies than we presently have. The inheritable hypohedonia could be checked by monozygotic-dizygotic twin studies and foster child studies, given a psychometric or psychophysiological "pleasure measure" of high validity. But the conjectured causal chain would presumably require follow-up studies of infants whose early developmental stages revealed normal emergency affectivity but a hedonic defect nevertheless – a tough measurement problem indeed!

I conclude by admitting ruefully that the clinical implications of these theoretical conjectures, are, at present, almost wholly negative. One justification for this communication is to set some good clinical brains working on constructive suggestions for the therapeutic management of patients whose complaints arise largely from their having inherited a defective hedonic capacity. The negative clinical implication is, of course, that interview tactics predicated upon the impedance view of all maladjustment are in such cases contraindicated for the simple reason that they take time and money, yet are unlikely to work.

My positive suggestions are, I am afraid, largely cognitive as well as tentative. I think people with low hedonic capacity should pay greater attention to the "hedonic bookkeeping" of their activities than would be necessary for people located midway or high on the hedonic capacity continuum. That is, it matters more to someone cursed with an inborn hedonic defect whether he is efficient and sagacious in selecting friends, jobs, cities, tasks, hobbies, and activities in general. Secondly, I have a strong clinical impression that, at least in the American culture, many people develop a kind of "secondary guilt" or shame about hedonic defects, particularly in the interpersonal domain, because the dominant ethos prescribes that everybody must be an extravert and must receive tremendous gratification from social interaction. I am convinced that active therapeutic maneuvers of the rational-emotive type (Ellis, 1962, 1971; Ellis & Harper, 1961) can be highly effective in reducing this secondary guilt and shame by helping the patient accept the fact that not everybody gets a big "kick" out of social interaction; there is no compelling reason why everybody has to be the same in this respect, any more than we all have to be the same in our needs for exercise, food, play, sleep, sexual outlet, music, poetry, art, beer, or whatever. But I must confess, again speaking conjecturally, that I have more faith in the ultimate efficacy of a psychopharmacological approach to this problem than I do in psychological intervention. Judging from what Freud had to say about the ultimate biochemical approach to constitutional issues, I believe he would probably go along with this suggestion.

REFERENCES

Brady, J.V. and Conrad, D.G. (1960). Some effects of limbic system self-stimulation upon conditioned emotional behavior. *J. Comp. Physiol. Psychol.*, 53:128-37.

Bunge, M.A.. (Ed). (1964). *The Critical Approach to Science and Philosophy: Essays in Honor of Karl R. Popper*. New York: Free Press.

Cattell, R.B. (1935). Perseveration and personality: Some experiments and a hypothesis. *J. Ment. Sci.*, 81:151-167.

Cattell, R.B. (1957). *Personality and Motivation Structure and Measurement.* Yonkers- on-Hudson, N.Y.: World Book Co.

Ellis, A. (1962). *Reason and Emotion in Psychotherapy*. New York: Lyle Stuart.

Ellis, A. (Ed.) (1971). *Growth Through Reason: Verbatim Cases in Rational-Emotive Therapy*. Palo Alto, Calif.: Science & Behavior Books.

Ellis, A. and Harper, R.A. (1961). *A Guide to Rational Living.* Englewood Cliffs, N.J.: Prentice-Hall.

English, H.B. and English, A.C. (1958). *A Comprehensive Dictionary of Psychological and Psychoanalytical Terms: A Guide to Usage*. New York: Longmans, Green & Co..

Escalona, S. (1968). *The Roots of Individuality*. Chicago: Aldine.

Farber, I.E. (1948). Response fixation under anxiety and non-anxiety conditions. *J. Exp. Psychol.*, 38:111-131.

Ferster, C.B. and Skinner, B.F. (1957) *Schedules of Reinforcement.* New York: Appleton-Century-Crofts.

Hernandez-Peon, R. (1966). Attention, sleep, motivation and behavior. In P. Bakon (Ed.), *Attention*. Princeton: D. van Nostrand.

Jones, M.C. (1924). Elimination of children's fears. *J. Exp. Psychol.*, 7:382-390.

Lieblich, I. and Olds, J. (1971). Selection for the readiness to respond to electrical stimulation of the hypothalamus as a reinforcing agent. *Brain Res.*, 27:153-161.

Marchand, W.E. (1961). Analgesic effect of masturbation. *Arch. Gen. Psychiatry*, 4:137- 138.

Meehl, P.E. (1962a). Schizotaxia, schizotypy, schizophrenia. *Am. Psychol.*, 17:827-838.

Meehl, P.E. (1962b). Psychopathology and purpose. In P. Hoch and J. Zubin (Eds.), *The Future of Psychiatry*. New York: Grune & Stratton.

Meehl, P.E. (1964). *Manual for Use with Checklist of Schizotypic Signs*. Minneapolis: Psychiatry Research Unit, University of Minnesota Medical School.

Meehl, P.E. (1970). Some methodological reflections on the difficulties of psychoanalytic research. In M. Radner and S. Winokur (Eds.), *Minnesota Studies in Philosophy of Science*, Vol. IV. Minneapolis: University of Minnesota Press.

Meehl, P.E. (1972a). Specific genetic etiology, psychodynamics, and therapeutic nihilism. *Int. J. Ment. Health*, 1:10-27.

Meehl, P.E. (1972b). A critical afterword. In I.I. Gottesman and J. Shields (Eds.), *Schizophrenia and Genetics: A Twin Study Vantage Point*, New York: Academic Press.

Meehl, P.E. (1974-75). Genes and the unchangeable core. *Voices: The Art and Science of Psychotherapy*, 10:25-35.

Meehl, P.E., Lykken, D.T., Schofield, W. and Tellegen, A. (1971). Recaptured-item technique (RIT): A method for reducing somewhat the subjective element in factor naming. *J. Exp. Res. Pers.*, 5:171-190.

Modell, W. (1961). *Relief of Symptoms*, Ed. 2. St. Louis: Mosby.

Olds, J. (1958). Studies of neuropharmacologicals by electrical and chemical manipulation of the brain in animals with chronically implanted electrodes. In P. B. Bradley (Ed.), *International Congress of Neuro-Psychopharmacology Proceedings*.

Popper, K.R. (1959). *The Logic of Scientific Discovery*. New York: Basic Books.

Popper, K.R. (1962). *Conjectures and Refutations*. New York: Basic Books.

Popper, K.R. (1972). *Objective Knowledge*. London: Oxford University Press.

Rado, S. (1956). *Psychoanalysis of Behavior: Collected Papers*. New York: Grune & Stratton.

Reid, L.D. (1973). Processes of fear reduction in systematic desensitization: An addendum to Wilson and Davison (1971). *Psychol. Bull.*, 79:107-109.

Schilpp, P.A., (Ed.). (1974). *The Philosophy of Karl Popper*. LaSalle, Ill.: Open Court Pub. Co.

Schofield, W. (1964). *Psychotherapy: The Purchase of Friendship*. Englewood Cliffs, N.J.: Prentice-Hall.

Williams, R.J. (1956). *Biochemical Individuality*. New York: Wiley.

Wilson, G.T. and Davison, G.C. (1971). Processes of fear reduction in systematic desensitization: Animal studies. *Psychol. Bull.*, 76:1-14.

Wolpe, J. and Lazarus, A. (1966). *Behavior Therapy Techniques: A Guide to the Treatment of Neuroses*, Elmsford, New York: Pergamon.

4

"Hedonic Capacity" Ten Years Later: Some Clarifications

PAUL E. MEEHL

Perhaps due to infelicitous formulations plus some bad editorial changes, and readers' familiarity with the emphasis on Rado's theory of schizotypy in earlier writings of mine, the intent of my "Hedonic Capacity: Some Conjectures" chapter has been variously misunderstood. I take this opportunity to offer some clarifying remarks, together with an expansion of a methodological point that was presented, but not defended, in a single sentence of the original paper.

The main point of the paper was the conjecture that while classical psychodynamics is largely correct in holding that pleasure is impaired in neurotic persons by the interference of anxiety as a state variable, as well as chronically by the anxiety signal putting the various defense mechanisms into operation, thereby inhibiting both the pleasure experience and the instrumental behaviors that tend statistically to bring it about (all of which I subsumed under the term "impedance theory"), we should consider another situation in which the causal relation between anxiety and hypohedonia is in precisely the opposite direction, namely, that a *primary (genetic) defect* in hedonic capacity results in an inadequate buffering or softening of aversive experiences. If this were true in some subset of our population, the exaggeration – both in degree and pervasiveness over life domains – of predominately aversive control which is so characteristic of the neurotic personality would be, in such cases, due to their basic deficiency in hedonic capacity.

It seemed to me that in addition to being of considerable theoretical importance in our general picture of the mind, such a possibility – which I believe is supported by one's clinical experience, once the clinician's mind is open to considering it as an option, rather than routinely asking what is being defended against or how is anxiety impeding pleasure – is of clinical importance. Pursuit in the therapeutic sessions of how the neurotic warding off is at work will be feckless if what is actually involved is an insufficient pleasure factor adequate to countervail anxiety. In addition to wasting time, and pushing interpretations that mobilize "realistic resistance," such pursuit has an opportunity cost, because hypohedonic clients need to learn this psychological fact as found differentially in life sectors, and to develop techniques for living within a "scarcity economy of pleasure," as Rado put it. (Hypohedonia leading to insufficient anxiety-softening might also be true for the other emergency affect, rage, and its attenuated forms of chronic anger, resentment, rejection of close relations and the like.) I was simply inviting clinician readers to open their minds to this interesting possibility, and to consult their clinical experience as to whether it seems to fit at least some cases.

I took it for granted, of course, that many different factors can keep people from having pleasure experiences, including an external situation which is thin on delivery of reinforcements and opportunities for need gratification. But I suggested that just as an external reinforcement schedule, defined by a patient's "social Skinner Box," may provide him with very little pleasure, an equivalent low-reward schedule *as subjectively experienced* could be produced by a biological deficiency.

I tried to emphasize, but apparently not clearly enough, that I thought of this reduced hedonic capacity not as a *pathological taxon* but as a *normal range individual differences variable*. I conceive the "pleasure parameter" as a disposition existing in all degrees from very low to very high, presumably polygenically determined, and in this respect quite analogous to other normal range non-pathological individual differences variables such as the general intelligence factor, the various components of mechanical ability, anxiety proneness, rage readiness, energy level, social introversion, and the numerous other temperamental factors, known and unknown, on which human beings differ one from another. My choice of the term "hedonic" (rather than Rado's "anhedonia") was meant to highlight the conception of a positive attribute, a power or disposition, manifesting itself in degrees. So the "deficiency" is merely being at the low end of this dimension. "Capacity" has the same flavor (as contrasted with "defect," "impairment," or the like). Also "capacity" connotes, in traditional trait theory and psychometrics, a second order disposition having a heritable component.

Due to my references to Rado's ideas and my earlier writings on schizophrenia, some correspondents have taken it that I consider anhedonia a more or less schizospecific trait, but the article in question does not say so, and I do not believe this. The relationship of hedonic impairment to schizoidia is in my opinion one of a polygenic modifier (I prefer for certain reasons to call it a potentiator instead of a modifier), influencing the probability of developing a clinical schizophrenia in a person who is genetically schizotypal. While I'm inclined to agree with Rado that this particular potentiater is a relatively important one, it is by no means confined to schizophrenia, being found also in persons with a kind of chronic, low grade non-cyclothymic depression, and, as Rado said in his later work, also quite frequent in the obsessional character.

The article attempted to pull together data from a variety of fact domains (e.g., animal learning, neurophysiology, factor analysis of clinical ratings) and I made no pretense to a rigorous showing of their equivalence; hence my title "Conjectures."

I have received correspondence about the article's expression of pessimism concerning the difficulty of separating primary hypohedonia from secondary pleasure impairment, and here I should explain the philosophy of science in which I operate. Suppose one is a strict operationist about concepts, and a strict verificationist about statements or theories (or those statement collections we call theories), and combines this with the social scientist's usual reliance upon statistical significance tests as a way of confirming theories. On those methodological views, it seems natural to say that if Meehl claims there is something called "primary hypohedonia," and something else that we find in the adult acculturated specimen, after his complex learning history, called "secondary anhedonia," such a theory is irresponsible if the theorist does not tell us, *right now*, how to tell them apart. But since I am neither an operationist nor a verificationist (positions having been held by no philosopher of science since roughly 50 years ago!) and I have grave doubts about the way in which significance tests are used in psychology to prove substantive theories, this complaint does not distress me. The fact of the matter is that many theories at a given stage of scientific knowledge are not strongly testable at the time they are proposed, and the history of the other sciences provides numerous examples. Of course a theorist can take advantage of this unfortunate fact of the unequal development of theories, required auxiliary theories, and instrumentation, to propound conjectures irresponsibly, but I hope I am not doing that. I made a couple of suggestions about ways to study primary pleasure deficit in very young children, but not being a child clinician or developmental psychologist I did not feel competent to discuss that in any detail. It is simply a fact that the human mind is complicated, and that it has a certain developmental and structural "layer" character, so that until more is known about the function of those brain centers involved in positive reinforcement (and, on the subjective side, in the pleasure experience) than we now know, and better psychometric or experimental devices are available, we cannot reliably distinguish primary from secondary hypohedonia. When you deal with a 25-year-old schizoid personality who experiences very little pleasure, it is difficult to design an experiment or build a psychometric instrument that will tell you whether he doesn't experience pleasure mostly because he's too angry and afraid to do so, or that he doesn't experience pleasure mainly because he has too few hedonic polygenes, that being one reason that he has so much anger and anxiety, these negative affects not being adequately softened by countervailing pleasure tone.

Conceiving hedonic capacity as a *dimensional higher-order disposition of polygenic origin* (analogous to Spearman's g) does not, of course, preclude the further possibility that some "pathological" cases occur on the basis of a developmental anomaly or a major genetic locus. As an analogy, I point out that the main heritable component of the general intelligence factor over "normal range individual differences in IQ" is polygenic is quite compatible with the existence of the Mendelizing mental deficiencies.

Finally, with regard to my reference to Olds (+) reinforcement centers, I thought it was interesting that there are inherited differences among rats in this respect. Being strongly hereditarian in my views about personality, I take it as obvious that any time a major individual differences variable is identifiable either clinically or psychometrically in human beings, some considerable causal component underlying that variation is genetic in origin. Minnesota colleagues have said I shouldn't have so readily identified the pleasure experience with the behavioral fact of reinforcement (defined as an event that produces an increase in operant strength); I of course agree with them that no such immediate automatic identification of the two is permissible. But it is inconceivable to me that, although conceptually distinct, they should not be intimately related.

5

Anhedonia, Hypohedonia and Pleasure Capacity in Major Depressive Disorders

DAVID C. CLARK
JAN FAWCETT

Good clinicians disagree about which clinical phenomena define the essence of anhedonia. This should be apparent from the great diversity of patients and phenomena discussed in this volume devoted to the problem of anhedonia. Some clinicians focus on the bland, blunt or flattened affective quality of many chronically ill psychiatric patients. Some focus on the unimaginative, excessively concrete and literal thinking styles of many patients and normals. Some focus on the lifelong, consistent behavior of those less engaged in social or recreational activities than most of the population. And others focus on the complaints of those who have acutely, temporarily lost their ability to enjoy accustomed pleasures. At the present time there is no empirical basis for estimating the degree of congruence or overlap among these differing definitions. Thus it should come as no surprise that anhedonia has been related to schizophrenia, depression, endogenous depression, neurotic conflict, narcissistic personality disorder, borderline personality disorder, post-traumatic states, alexithymia and normal individual differences by leading theoreticians at different points in time.

One solution to this confusion of nomenclature arrives lies in the operational definition of each investigator's concept of anhedonia. Operational definitions allow other investigators to test the replicability of clinical research findings and evaluate the congruence among different definitions of anhedonia. Only when differing definitions of anhedonia are reconciled with one another will it be possible to clarify the relationship between anhedonia and different psychopathological states.

Our work on anhedonia has been strongly influenced by the clinical theories of two leading theoreticians: Paul Meehl and Donald Klein. Meehl (See Chapter 3, this volume) was the first to discuss the possibility that anhedonia represents a variation of normal character organization. He postulated that in many patients who seek professional help, there is an inborn feebleness of physiologic positive reinforcers that normally function as modulators of aversive life conditions. These patients function at the low end of a normally distributed continuum of "basic hedonic capacity." Persons at the low end of this continuum are less prepared to buffer aversive life conditions with their own experiences of pleasure (remembered or anticipated), and are therefore more vulnerable to developing psychopathology than others. Meehl's position encourages us to think in terms of "hypohedonia" and "hyperhedonia" as characterological features, where we are more accustomed to think of "anhedonia" as a pathological state easily distinguished from normalcy.

Meehl's hypothesis stands in stark contrast to the clinical theory of anhedonic phenomena published by Klein and colleagues (1974, 1980) about the same time. Klein assigned preeminence to pleasure capacity as a symptom for classifying patients with major depression. Reviewing an accumulation of factor analytic studies of the symptoms of depressed patients, Klein suggested that anhedonia represents a marker for classical ("endogenomorphic") depression states. He hypothesized that anhedonic depressions (i.e., those characterized by consummatory pleasure deficit in addition to appetitive pleasure deficit) are associated with a specific functional disorder of the central nervous system, and show a more favorable response to treatment with tricyclic antidepressant medication than do other types of major depression. Furthermore, Klein observed that the capacity to experience pleasure returns before other depressive symptoms show improvement in patients recovering from classical depression states. Klein's definition of the "endogenomorphic" syndrome has been adapted for use in the DSM-III classification scheme, where "melancholia" is essentially a major depression characterized by a pervasive non-reactive anhedonic state. There has been at least one rigorous empirical test of the internal validity of the "melancholia" syndrome (Young, Scheftner, et al., 1986), and those results tend to support Klein's position.

Thus Meehl and Klein offer the clinician two distinctly different ways to conceptualize the anhedonia of a depressed patient. Meehl would encourage us to consider the possibility that anhedonia represents a lifelong characterological trait, and perhaps a characterological vulnerability predisposing the patient to depressive decompensations under conditions of adversity. Klein would encourage us to consider the possibility that anhedonia, subclassified according to the manifestations of appetitive or consummatory pleasure deficit, represents an illness state associated with a distinct subtype of depression. Meehl would lead us to expect that the patient will continue to show himself anhedonic after complete recovery from the depressive illness. Klein would lead us to expect that the patient will regain his premorbid pleasure capacity after complete recovery from the depressive illness.

In a series of preliminary studies (Fawcett, Clark et al., 1983a; Fawcett, Clark et al., 1983b; Clark, Fawcett et al., 1984), we examined the relationship between individual pleasure capacity and depressive state over brief periods of time to test some of the clinical theories of Meehl and Klein. Initially, we designed a patient self-report scale to measure momentary pleasure capacity. The Fawcett-Clark Pleasure Capacity Scale (FCPCS) asks subjects to imagine the degree of their pleasurable response to a variety of normally enjoyable situations and describe each response on a five-point scale. Our results (Fawcett, Clark et al., 1983a) showed that the FCPCS demonstrates good internal consistency, and item responses were distributed along a single latent continuum, supporting the hypothesis that the scale items tap a unidimensional rather than a multidimensional construct. There was no basis for distinguishing between different "types" of pleasure (e.g., physical versus social). Sexual intimacy, marital affection, and the opportunity to enjoy the well-being of grown offspring were consistently the most highly valued situations for all subjects, regardless of diagnosis.

When we examined the concurrent validity of the FCPCS (Fawcett, Clark et al., 1983a), we found that pleasure capacity scores correlated significantly with indices of depression (-.46), social impairment (-.39), anhedonia as assessed by Chapman's (Chapman and Raulin, 1976) Anhedonia Scale (-.42), hopelessness (-.27) and extraversion (+.28). Pleasure capacity scores did not correlate significantly with age, sex, indices of neuroticism, IQ or abstraction ability. In a separate study of the response to amphetamine challenge in 62 outpatients with major depression (DSM-III criteria), we also showed that the antidepressant and pleasure-enhancing effects of the drug are associated with different time courses (Clark, Edwards et al., unpublished manuscript).

We found that 18% of psychiatric in-patients with major depression (DSM-III criteria), but no manic, schizoaffective or schizophrenic inpatient exhibited FCPCS scores falling below the lowest-ranging score for psychiatrically healthy subjects (Fawcett, Clark et al., 1983a). A mixture analysis divided all depressed patients' FCPCS scores into two distinct distributions: one that corresponded to the distribution exhibited by psychiatrically well subjects (encompassing 88% of the depressed patients); and one that was extremely anhedonic (encompassing the remaining 12% of depressed patients). We concluded that the data provide some justification for distinguishing between two subtypes of depression: one characterized by extreme anhedonia, and another characterized by a normal-range capacity for pleasureable experiences.

The majority of depressed patients (88%) gave responses suggesting that their pleasure capacity was normal or intact despite the superimposed depressive illness. Only a minority (12%) of depressed patients really lost most or all of their capacity to imagine or recall their own pleasureable experiences. These observations do not shed any light on fluctuations in pleasure capacity over the course of a depressive episode for patients in either group, or on the fate of anhedonia after recovery from depression.

In response to our results, Klein has suggested that the anhedonic phenomena assessed by the FCPCS represents an appetitive rather than a consummatory pleasure deficit, because the scale is based on patient self-report to imaginary situations (see Chapter 1 in this volume). We purposefully designed scale items that invite the subject to respond passively to pleasurable situations remote in time and presented under fictional or ideal circumstances in order to encourage reactivity, without asking the subject to deny the severity of current depressive symptoms. Klein himself explicitly hypothesized (Klein, 1974) that "endogenomorphic" depressed patients cannot experience pleasure from current sensory input, and show a decreased ability to respond affectively to pleasurable imagery by means of recollection or anticipation. Furthermore, FCPCS items that were defined a priori as appetitive or consummatory in quality loaded together on the same single dimension in item reliability analyses (Fawcett, Clark et al., 1983a). All these observations lead us to reserve judgement on the essentially appetitive or consummatory nature of the FCPCS. Clearly studies comparing patient self-report scores with behavioral observations, the report of collateral informants, and expert clinical judgements will clarify the appetitive or consummatory nature of the FCPCS with the necessary and sufficient kinds of evidence.

Supposing for the moment that we may be able to identify two distinct subtypes of depressed patients with the aid of the FCPCS, we went on to examine sociodemographic, clinical, and outcome differences between the two subtypes (Fawcett, Clark et al., 1983b). Extremely anhedonic depressives were more severely depressed and hopeless, less neurotic, younger and more likely to be female than normally hedonic depressives. The two groups did not differ, however, in terms of delusions, hallucinations, suicidal ideation, psychomotor retardation, or length of hospital stay. Klein had previously hypothesized (1974) that endogenomorphic depressives are more profoundly depressed and less neurotic than other depressives, which was supported by our results. He also hypothesized that endogenomorphic patients are older, which ran contrary to our results.

Higher scores on a cluster of six symptom items from the Beck Depression Inventory were associated with the anhedonic subtype: loss of social interest, loss of appetite, loss of sexual interest, loss of satisfaction, work inhibition, and suicidal tendencies. The first five symptoms are clearly consistent with the clinical concept of anhedonia. Higher scores on a cluster of four other Beck items were associated with the normally hedonic subtype: pessimism, indecision, irritability, and hypochondriasis.

To examine the course associated with each depressive subtype, we prospectively followed groups of anhedonic and normally hedonic inpatients from index hospitalization through hospital discharge and a seven-month follow-up (Clark, Fawcett et al., 1984). Patients who were initially subtyped as "anhedonic" persisted in evidencing significantly lower FCPCS scores than other depressives at discharge and seven-month follow-up, even when the comparison was limited to patients fully recovered from their depressive illness. Anhedonic depressives were more severely depressed on hospital admission, showed a more rapid rate of symptom improvement during the first weeks of inpatient treatment, and showed a greater incidence of complete clinical recovery at the seven-month follow-up; yet they were still significantly more anhedonic than other depressed patients after recovery. The better treatment response to antidepressants shown by the anhedonic group is again consistent with Klein's clinical theory.

It is possible to think that the observed association between anhedonic-subtype depressive illness and greater likelihood of clinical recovery at seven-month follow-up might be mediated by the personality trait of neuroticism. In several studies of acutely depressed patients (Kerr, Schapira et al., 1970; Paykel, Klerman et al., 1974; Weissman, Prusoff et al., 1978), the only demographic or clinical variable significantly related to outcome was neuroticism; high neuroticism scores were associated with poor long-term outcome. Since normally hedonic subtype depressed patients are significantly more neurotic than their anhedonic counterparts, it might be that their higher initial neuroticism scores are the sole explanation for their worse outcome. Therefore we compared the contributions of FCPCS and neuroticism scores (as assessed by the Eysenck Brief Inventory) (Eysenck and Eysenck, 1964) to outcome variance in a multivariate analysis. Both variables emerged as significant and independent predictors of clinical recovery (Fawcett, Clark et al., 1983b).

In sum, the results of a series of studies using the FCPCS to operationally define pleasure capacity provide some justification for conceptualizing the anhedonia manifested by a minority of depressed patients as a characterological trait that continues to be present after complete clinical recovery from depression. This position is most consistent with Meehl's, rather than Klein's, clinical theory. It is not clear whether the anhedonic depressives were anhedonic *prior* to the onset of their depressive episodes in our studies, however, because they were selected for study after they had been admitted to a psychiatric hospital for depression.

Two more recent studies have allowed us to take a preliminary look at data bearing on the relationship between low pleasure capacity and the incidence of depressive illness or impaired work functioning in normal (i.e., non-patient) subjects. In the first study (Clark, Salazar-Grueso et al., 1984), we assessed fifty-five interns from one university medical center at the beginning of their work year, and again six months later using structured interviews and Research Diagnostic Criteria (Spitzer, Endicott et al., 1977). Fifteen interns (27%) developed a depressive syndrome at some point during the six-month period, an incidence rate similar to the one reported by Valko and Clayton (1975) nine years earlier at another university medical center. In our sample, parental history of depression and high scores on trait neuroticism were significantly associated with onset of depression, but low capacity for experiencing pleasure (at initial assessment), personal history of psychopathology, and absolute workload were not.

In a second study (Clark, Morrison et al., 1984), we collected data on pleasure capacity and depressive symptoms from eighty-eight senior executive officers of Fortune 500 companies, and compared these scores with independent ratings of work functioning and success. The 11% of executives with serious work-related problems showed no more depression than the rest, but did show significantly *higher* FCPCS scores. These results are exactly opposite from those we predicted at the outset of the study. Individual differences in pleasure capacity were not associated with greater or less success for the 89% of executives evidencing no work-related impairment. After a review of individual interview data with each subject, we hypothesized that the relatively high FCPCS scores of the least successful executives reflect a defensive process of denial or reaction formation rather than an excessively joyful personality trait.

Thus we find no evidence as yet for concluding that anhedonic individuals are more vulnerable to depressive illness states or impaired work functioning than other people. Our observations are restricted to an extremely small number of normal subjects, however. One might expect that a sample of distinctly anhedonic "normal" subjects would only emerge through screening and comparing hundreds or thousands of normals. One might also expect that if Meehl's portrayal of the characterological fragility of the anhedonic individual is accurate, then relatively few anhedonics are likely to show the resourcefulness and stamina necessary to become the medical students or senior executive officers at Fortune 500 companies that we have studied.

One of us (DCC) is studying several samples of medical students longitudinally from the first day of medical school, creating an opportunity to examine the construct validity of pleasure capacity as defined by the FCPCS. Students are serially assessed by a fixed battery of survey and projective instruments, allowing us to characterize them and map changes over time on dimensions of sociodemographic background, mood, attitude, personality, social involvement, academic performance, alcohol and illicit drug use (Clark, Eckenfels et al., 1985; Clark, Daugherty et al., 1986; Zeldow, Clark et al., 1985a; Zeldow, Clark et al., 1985b). Preliminary results from the medical student studies suggest that pleasure capacity shows a consistent low-order correlation with mood-related variables such as depression and self-esteem, but a more substantial correlation with two personality measures of emotional expressivity: femininity and intimacy motivation. Higher FCPCS scores are correlated with higher femininity and intimacy scores.

Femininity, as assessed by the Personality Attributes Questionnaire (Spence, Helmreich et al., 1974) is defined by items considered socially desirable in both sexes but that females are believed to possess in greater abundance than males (e.g., gentleness, expressiveness, agreeableness, and concern for others). Intimacy motivation was assessed from imaginative stories given in response to each of five TAT pictures using a thematic coding system developed by McAdams (1980, 1982). Intimacy motivation is apparent in a greater readiness to perceive and elaborate on warm, close and caring interpersonal relationships in story responses.

Thus preliminary findings that FCPCS scores are significantly correlated with the personality traits of femininity and intimacy – personality traits that typically show a high degree of intra-subject reliability over time – suggest that the construct of pleasure capacity has at least one narrowly defined social implication. Individuals high in pleasure capacity tend to be emotionally expressive and concerned with close, caring relationships. Those low in hedonic capacity may operate at a distinct disadvantage: they are less communicative and less embedded in close, caring social relationships.

The etiology of the anhedonic states and the normal variations in pleasure capacity we have discussed remain unclear. Both Meehl (Chapter 3, this volume) and Krystal (Chapter 7, this volume; 1978) have discussed possible etiologies of characterological anhedonia and the clinical problems encountered by individuals so afflicted. Meehl postulated a normally distributed continuum of basic hedonic capacity, and Krystal has interpreted the anhedonia of some patients as the residue of a prior traumatic state. It is also possible that the anhedonia we observe in some patients represents an irreversible global diminution of affective capacity, such as that postulated in cases of alexithymia (Sifneos, 1967). Sifneos has suggested that all alexithymic patients exhibit anhedonic features, whereas only some patients evidencing anhedonia are alexithymic (see Chapter 8, this volume). If Sifneos is right, then the global affective responsivity of a patient must be assessed before the narrower conclusion of a pleasure capacity deficit can be drawn.

In our clinical work, we have been impressed with the perspective offered by attribution analysis (Jones, Kanouse et al., 1972; Weiner, 1972; Harvey, Ickes et al., 1976) for structuring brief therapy with some patients complaining of anhedonia in the absence of a major depressive illness. Attribution analysis is concerned with an individual's mental representation of the world and the manner by which the individual interprets personal experience. The focus of attribution analysis is largely cognitive, but it has clear definable affective and behavioral implications as well.

Attribution analysis might classify anhedonic manifestations as falling into one of three categories, related to: (a) expectations; (b) evaluation of failure or success; and (c) sources of pleasure. The assumption underlying each category is an etiological one. The first two categories imply some attributional error, rooted in experience, that can be altered in therapy. The third category implies a deficit that may be conceived as either inborn or acquired in some very fundamental sense.

With regard to *expectations*, any life event is represented by the individual affected in attributional terms; that is, the event imbued with characteristics and properties based on past experiences and generalizations from comparable events. The sum of these attributions may be considered a set of expectations concerning the potential for action and pleasure inherent to the event. Thus, individuals may fail to recognize the potential for pleasure in many kinds of situations because they have not accumulated sufficient pleasurable life experiences, or because their past experience hinders the development of appropriate expectations for new events, or because they employ faulty logic to generate expectations.

With regard to *success evaluation*, all goal-directed activity produces feedback concerning outcome which the individual interprets as personal success or failure (i.e., is the goal reached or not?). Determination of success or failure, so closely associated with pleasureable or demoralized feedback responses, is nevertheless an extremely subjective attribution, especially with respect to the causes of success or failure. While it is adaptive in most situations to assign responsibility for success or failure correctly and develop the resulting capacity for corrective action, people usually blame their failures on external circumstances, and take personal credit for successes. This attributional bias may be reversed for some depressed and anhedonic patients. The correct assessment of causality in success or failure experiences helps counteract failure with corrective action, facilitating ultimate success and the pleasure associated with goal achievement. For the discouraged patient experiencing little pleasure, better or correct attribution combats an acquired sense of learned helplessness and encourages the individual to be an active agent searching for pleasure, rather than a passive recipient of mundane experience and disappointments.

With regard to *sources of pleasure*, it is possible that some individuals may be unable to access pleasureable experiences for inborn biological (as postulated by Meehl and Sifneos) or characterological (as postulated by Krystal) reasons. It is also possible that some individuals do not come to regard the experience of pleasure as consistent with their sense of selfhood. For these latter individuals, the process of firming or strengthening the self may be directly opposed to the process of cultivating the capacity to experience pleasure. For some there may be a deep-seated fear that the experience of pleasure will decompose a fragile or carefully compiled self.

The three categories defined by our attribution analysis suggest a series of questions that may guide the clinical interviewer or investigator attempting to achieve a more refined understanding of the anhedonic quality of a given patient: (1) What set of expectations does the patient bring to activities and life events that might mediate his/her hedonic responsivity?; (2) How high of a threshold does the patient maintain for evaluating personal successes, and how does the patient assign cause or responsibility for failure experiences?; and (3) Does the patient evidence any rudimentary capacity for pleasure? Is there any evidence for non-conscious or subconscious defense against experiences of pleasure?

In conclusion, the data suggest there is an enduring trait-like quality to the construct of pleasure capacity as we have operationally defined that construct. A small minority of hospitalized depressed patients appear to be anhedonic, and distinctly different enough from other depressed patients to warrant a subtype classification pending further research. Anhedonic depressives remain anhedonic even after complete recovery from their depressive illness. We have found no direct evidence that individuals lower in pleasure capacity are more susceptible to depressive illness, but we have observed that pleasure capacity is correlated with the personality traits of femininity and concern with intimacy. Femininity has been associated with greater liability to depressed mood and less likelihood of illicit drug involvement in our medical student samples (Zeldow, Clark et al., 1985a).

REFERENCES

Clark, D.C., Daugherty, S.R., Zeldow, P.B. et al. (1986). Alcohol use patterns of first-year medical students: II. Psychosocial characteristics associated with drinking level. *Alcoholism: Clinical and Experimental Research*, 10:65-70.

Clark, D.C., Eckenfels, E.J., Daugherty, S.R. et al. (1985). Alcohol use patterns of first year medical students: I. Development of shared norms. *Alcoholism: Clinical and Experimental Research*, 9:38-44.

Clark, D.C., Edwards, J., Fawcett, J. et al. (unpublished). Components of pathological mood: The responsivity of depressive mood and pleasure capacity to amphetamine challenge in depressed patients.

Clark, D.C., Fawcett, J., Salazar-Grueso, E. et al. (1984). Seven-month clinical outcome of anhedonic and normally hedonic depressed inpatients. *American Journal of Psychiatry*, 141:1216-1220.

Clark, D.C., Morrison, D.E., Fawcett, J. (1984). Is capacity for pleasure associated with executive career success? *Journal of Occupational Medicine*, 26:37-40.

Clark, D.C., Salazar-Grueso, E., Grabler, P. et al. (1984). Predictors of depression during the first six months of internship. *American Journal of Psychiatry*, 141:1095-1098.

Eysenck, S., Eysenck, H. (1964). An improved short questionnaire for the measurement of extraversion and neuroticism. *Life Sciences*, 3:1103-1109.

Fawcett, J., Clark, D.C., Scheftner, W.A. et al. (1983a). Assessing anhedonia in psychiatric patients: The Pleasure Scale. *Archives of General Psychiatry*, 40:79-84.

Fawcett, J., Clark, D.C., Scheftner, W.A. et al. (1983b). Differences between anhedonic and normally hedonic depressive states. *American Journal of Psychiatry*, 140:1027-1030.

Harvey, J.H., Ickes, W.J., Kidd, R.F. (editors) (1976). *Directions in Attribution Research, Volume I*. Hillsdale, N.J., Erlbaum Associates.

Jones, E.E., Kanouse, D.E., Kelly, H.H. et al. (1972). *Attribution: Perceiving the Causes of Behavior*. Morriston, N.J., General Learning Press.

Kerr, T., Schapira, K., Roth, M. et al. (1970). The relationship between the Maudsley Personality Inventory and the course of affective disorders. *British Journal of Psychiatry*, 116:11-19.

Klein, D.F. (1974). Endogenomorphic depression: A conceptual and terminological revision. *Archives of General Psychiatry*, 31:447-454.

Klein, D.F. Gittelman, R., Quitkin, F. et al. (1980). *Diagnosis and Drug Treatment of Psychiatric Disorders: Adults and Children.* Baltimore, Williams & Wilkins Co.

Krystal, H. (1978). Trauma and affects. *Psychoanalytic Study of the Child*, 33:81-116.

McAdams, D.P. (1980). A thematic coding system for the intimacy motive. *Journal of Research in Personality*, 14:413-432.

McAdams, D.P. (1982). Experiences of intimacy and power: Relationships between social motives and autobiographical memory. *Journal of Personality and Social Psychology*, 42:292-302.

Paykel, E., Klerman, G., Prusoff, B. (1974). Prognosis of depression and the endogenous-neurotic distinction. *Psychological Medicine*, 4:57-64.

Sifneos, P.E. (1967). Clinical observations on some patients suffering from a variety of psychosomatic disorders. *Proceedings of the Seventh European Conference on Psychoso matic Research.* Basel, Karger.

Spence, J.T., Helmreich, R. L., Stapp, J. (1974). The Personality Attributes Questionnaire: A measure of sex-role stereotypes and masculinity-femininity. *JSAS Catalog of Selected Documents in Psychology*, 4:43.

Spitzer, R.L., Endicott, J., Robins, E. (1977). *Research Diagnostic Criteria for a Selected Group of Functional Disorders*, ed 3. New York, Biometrics Research Division, New York State Psychiatric Institute.

Valko, R., Clayton, P. (1975). Depression in the internship. *Diseases of the Nervous System*, 36:26-29.

Weiner, B. (1972). *Theories of Motivation: From Mechanism to Cognition.* Chicago, Markham.

Weissman, M.M., Prusoff, B.A., Klerman, G.L. (1978). Personality and the prediction of long-term outcome of depression. *American Journal of Psychiatry*, 135:797-800.

Young, M.A., Scheftner, W.A., Klerman, G.L. et al. (1986). The endogenous subtype of depression: A study of its internal construct validity. *British Journal of Psychiatry* 148:257-267.

Zeldow, P.B., Clark, D. C., Daugherty, S. R. (1985a). Masculinity, femininity, type A behavior and psychosocial adjustment in medical students. *Journal of Personality and Social Psychology*, 48:481-492.

Zeldow, P.B., Clark, D.C., Daugherty, S.R. et al. (1985b). Personality indicators of psychosocial adjustment in first-year medical students. *Social Science and Medicine*, 20:95-100.

6

Negative Symptoms, Affective Deficit States, and Intellectual Dysfunction in Chronic Schizophrenia

*MICHAEL F. POGUE-GEILE AND MARTIN HARROW**

Historically, affective deficits have been considered as among the most important aspects of schizophrenia. Kraepelin (1919), when he first defined the syndrome, wrote that the "common characteristic of (dementia praecox) is a peculiar destruction of the internal connections of the psychic personality, the effects of (which) predominate in the emotional and volitional spheres of mental life" (p. 3). Similarly, Bleuler (1950) also designated a deficit in "affectivity" as one of his fundamental symptoms of schizophrenia. Despite this early importance ascribed to affective deficits in schizophrenia, research on these topics has tended to languish until relatively recently.

Much of the more recent research on affective deficit in schizophrenia has investigated the broader construct of "negative symptoms" (Andreasen, 1979a; 1982; Crow, 1980, 1982; Fish, 1962; Huber, Gross et al., 1980; Pogue-Geile & Harrow, 1984a; Strauss, Carpenter et al., 1974; Wing, 1978; Wing & Brown, 1970). Negative symptoms have been respectively defined as "the relative absence of normal functioning" (Strauss, Carpenter et al., 1974), as characteristics of the schizophrenic defect state (Andreasen, 1982), and as deficit symptoms

* This research was supported, in part, by Grant MH-26341, from the National Institute of Mental Health, and Research Grants from the John D. and Catherine T. MacArthur Foundation, and the Carnegie Corporation. The authors also wish to thank Joanne Marengo, Ph.D., and Ilene Lanin-Kettering, Ph.D., for assisting in data collection.

(Chapman & Chapman, 1973). Such psychopathological deficits as flat affect, poverty of speech, and psychomotor retardation have traditionally been included within the negative symptom construct. Thus, the term "negative symptoms" is a broad concept that includes affective deficits such as flat affect, in addition to other behavioral and cognitive deficits. The present study is an investigation of this broad construct. Specifically, we examined negative symptoms in chronic schizophrenia and their relationships with other deficits in intellectual functioning.

In addition to the traditional negative symptoms of flat affect, poverty of speech and psychomotor retardation, subjectively experienced affective deficits such as anhedonia, which is discussed in other chapters of this volume, have also been included as negative symptoms by some theorists (e.g., Andreasen & Olsen, 1982). To date however the relationship between behavioral ratings of flat affect and self-reported affective deficits (e.g., anhedonia) has been little investigated. Although subjective anhedonia may prove to be an important negative symptom, the present research emphasized the other traditional behavioral ratings of affective deficit, such as flat affect, as one aspect of the negative symptom construct.

Negative symptoms are often contrasted with florid, "positive" symptoms which represent some behavioral excess that has a bizarre quality. Most positive symptoms involve a wealth of unusual thinking (Fish, 1962; Harrow & Quinlan, in press; Pogue-Geile & Harrow, 1984a). Symptoms such as delusions, hallucinations, and florid formal thought disorder are generally classified as positive symptoms (Strauss, Carpenter et al., 1974). This distinction between negative and positive symptoms was originally made by Hughlings Jackson (1887) as part of his evolutionary theory of the nervous system. Most recent writers have retained his descriptive terminology, but have generally eschewed his original physiological speculations.

Recent theorizing by Strauss, Carpenter, and Andreasen in this country and by Crow in Great Britain has attributed several putative characteristics to negative symptoms. Strauss, Carpenter et al., (1974) have hypothesized that negative symptoms, such as flat affect, should be relatively persistent and should be poor prognostic signs for later functioning. A number of investigators have also assumed that negative symptoms should be most frequent in older, chronic schizophrenics (e.g., Bridge, Cannon et al., 1978). During the acute phase, they hypothesize that positive symptoms will be fluctuating, with relatively little prognostic importance, and that they will have receded in importance in older, chronic schizophrenics.

An hypothesized biological basis for such putative differences between negative and positive symptoms has been recently proposed by Crow (1980, 1982) who has suggested that negative symptoms (his Type II syndrome) may be due to structural brain abnormalities, such as can be visualized on CT scan. In contrast, positive symptoms (Type I syndrome) are hypothesized to be due to some dysfunction in dopaminergic neural transmission. These two symptom syndromes are held to be independent processes within schizophrenia that may or may not co-occur. This position suggests that negative symptoms should be important in delineating a subgroup of schizophrenics characterized by intellectual deterioration, poor outcome, cortical atrophy on CT scan, and poor response to antipsychotic medication; in short, the "dementia" of dementia praecox (Crow, 1980; Johnstone, Crow et al., 1978).

The present research investigated this hypothesized association between negative symptoms and intellectual deficit in schizophrenia to determine whether the two do in fact tend to co-occur to form a dementia-like syndrome. In addition, the relationship between positive and negative symptoms was explored. Whereas Crow has suggested that positive and negative symptoms are independent syndromes, other investigators, such as Andreasen (Andreasen & Olsen, 1982) propose that the two are negatively related, or at opposite ends of a bipolar dimension. Our own research with an acute sample of schizophrenics has suggested that negative and positive symptoms are independent of one another (Pogue-Geile & Harrow, 1984a) but we have not investigated this issue in chronic schizophrenia. In addition, the notion that positive symptoms have declined in importance in chronic schizophrenia was investigated. These hypotheses were examined within a sample of chronic schizophrenics who might be considered at "high risk" for Crow's Type II negative symptoms syndrome.

METHOD

Subjects

This study is part of a program of longitudinal research, the Chicago Follow-up Study, which is studying both positive and negative symptoms in various phases of schizophrenia (Grinker & Harrow, in press; Harrow & Quinlan, in press). One major focus is an investigation of negative symptoms' specificity to schizophrenia, the correlates of negative symptoms (Pogue-Geile & Harrow, 1984a; 1984b; Pogue-Geile, Harrow et al., 1983), their prognostic importance

(Pogue-Geile, Harrow et al., 1984), and potential psychometric indices of negative symptoms (Pogue-Geile & Harrow, 1984; Rubin, Pogue-Geile et al., 1984).

The 54 schizophrenics who participated in this study were selected from current inpatients at a Chicago-area long-term state psychiatric hospital who had completed at least 10 years of education. Two subgroups of patients were selected. One, the "chronic" subgroup (N = 22), included patients who had been hospitalized at least eight of the last ten years. In addition, a "revolving door" subgroup (N = 32) was composed of patients who had their first hospitalization at least five years prior to assessment, with at least three separate readmissions since then (Harrow, Marengo et al., in press). As these subgroups did not differ in the analyses presented below, only the results for the combined total group will be reported. Patients were interviewed with a revised version of the Schedule for Affective Disorders and Schizophrenia (SADS) (Spitzer & Endicott, 1978), and based on this and their hospital chart, the patients were diagnosed, blind to other data, by a trained diagnostic team using the New Haven Schizophrenia Index (NHSI) (Astrachan, Harrow et al., 1972). Patients who met the NHSI criteria for schizophrenia at the time of their current hospital admission were selected for this study. All of these subjects also had a hospital diagnosis of schizophrenia and had been floridly psychotic (hallucinating and/or delusional) at some time during their current hospitalization.

Table 6.1 presents demographic data for the total sample of schizophrenics. The average age of the sample was 36 years old. Their average duration of disorder since first hospitalization was 14 years, with an average of nine years having been spent in psychiatric hospitals. The average educational level was generally low, with 44 percent of the patients having never finished high school. Almost all of the patients (95%) were taking antipsychotic medications at the time of assessment. As Table 6.1 shows, this is a sample of severely disturbed schizophrenics with a substantial prior history of serious difficulties.

MEASURES

The patients were assessed in the three general areas of: negative symptoms, intellectual functioning and positive symptoms.

Table 6.1
Demographic and Clinical Information

Demographic/Clinical Variable	Schizophrenics (N = 54)	
Sex (female)[1]	25	(46%)
Age[2]	36.1	(10.2)
Education[1]		
Not H.S. Graduate	24	(44%)
H.S. Graduate	23	(43%)
More than H.S.	7	(13%)
Age at First Hospitalization[2]	22.4	(8.0)
Years Since First Hospitalization[2]	13.6	(9.3)
Number of Previous Hospitalizations[2]	5.3	(5.0)
Lifetime Duration of Hospitalization (Months)[2]	109.4	(99.5)

1 – N (%)
2 – Means (standard deviation)

Negative Symptoms

The current assessment of negative symptoms and affective deficit focused on objective ratings of behavior using rating scales that we have successfully employed in our other research on negative symptoms (Pogue-Geile & Harrow, 1984a; 1984b; Pogue-Geile, Harrow et al., 1984). These negative symptoms scales were derived from the Behavior Rating Schedule of the Psychiatric Assessment Interview (PAI) (Carpenter, Sacks et al., 1976). The PAI is a modification by Strauss and Carpenter (1974) of the eighth edition of Wing's Present State Exam (PSE) (WHO, 1973). The ratings were based only on behavior shown during the assessment interview. Individual items were rated as either: 0) absent, 1) present but in mild form, or 2) present in marked form. These behavior ratings were made by trained interviewers who were blind to the hypotheses under study.

Items from the Behavior Rating Schedule of the PAI that were judged to index relevant negative symptoms were grouped to form three additive scales: Poverty of Speech, Flat Affect, and Psychomotor Retardation. In addition, we computed an overall Total Score that was a sum of the three individual scores. Table 6.2 presents the item

Table 6.2
Item Compostion of Negative Smptom Behavior Rating Scales

Poverty of Speech	Flat Affect
a. Long lapses before replying	a. Avoids looking at interviewer
b. Restriction of quantity speech	b. Blank, expressionless face
c. Patient fails to answer	c. Reduced emotion shown when emotional material discussed.
d. Speech slowed	d. Apathetic and uninterested
e. Blocking	e. Monotonous voice
	f. Low voice, difficult to hear
Psychomotor Retardation	
a. Slowed in movements	
b. Reduction in volun-tary movements	

Note: Items are from the Behavior Rating Inventory of the Psychiatric Assessment Interview (Stauss & Carpenter, 1974).

composition of each scale. The item content of these scales is a modification of that recently proposed by Andreasen (1981; 1982). However, the present scales are based only on behavior shown during the assessment interview and do not include information about functioning in other areas, such as employment or social relations. This approach allows us to empirically determine the relationship between clinically assessed symptomatology and functioning in other areas. Our flat affect scale also differs from Andreasen's scale in that we do not include inappropriate affect in our construct. Descriptively, inappropriate affect seems to differ from flat affect and therefore was not combined with it. We also do not include poverty of content as a negative symptom for similar reasons. The three scales were quite internally consistent as evidenced by the following Cronbach Alphas: Poverty of Speech, .64; Flat Affect, .75; Psychomotor Retardation, .48; and Total Score, .81. Inter-rater reliability of these scales was evaluated from videotapes of a separate sample of 20 patients. Intraclass correlations (ICC) between two independent raters were satisfactory; ICC = .88 for Poverty of Speech; ICC = .69 for Flat Affect; ICC = .67 for Psychomotor Retardation; and ICC = .87 for Total Score. The three scales were significantly intercorrelated as follows: r = .29 for Flat affect vs. Psychomotor Retardation, r = .51 for Poverty of Speech vs. Psychomotor Retardation, and r = .60 for Flat Affect vs. Poverty of Speech. Further details on the characteristics of these scales are available in Pogue-Geile and Harrow (1984a). Based on other research (Pogue-Geile & Harrow, 1984a) cutting scores of "2" or greater for the individual scales and scores of "4" or greater for the total score were used as criteria for the presence of definite negative symptoms.

Intellectual Functioning

Intellectual functioning in several different domains was assessed with three subtests from the Wechsler Adult Intelligence Scale (WAIS) (Wechsler, 1955). The Information subtest was used to determine the patients' long-term store of information. The Comprehension subtest provided a measure of social knowledge and norms, and the Digit Symbol Substitution Test (DSST), which is a timed copying test, was used as a measure of psychomotor speed.

Positive Symptoms

In addition to these measures of negative symptoms and intellectual functioning, three types of positive symptoms were also assessed. The presence of hallucinations and delusions of any type during the past month was rated from the SADS interview. Both of these symptoms were rated on a three point scale of: 1) absent; 2) mild or equivocal; and 3) definitely present.

The third positive symptom was positive formal thought disorder (Fish, 1962; Andreasen, 1979a) as indexed by our composite measure of bizarre-idiosyncratic thinking (Harrow & Quinlan, in press). Bizarre-idiosyncratic thinking includes most of the types of formal thought disorder described in the DSM-III, such as loose associations, derailment, and illogicality. Our composite measure was derived from the highest rating of bizarre-idiosyncratic thinking on either the Gorham Proverbs Test (Goldstein & Scheerer, 1941), or the Comprehension subtest of the Wechsler Adult Intelligence Scale (WAIS) (Wechsler, 1955). A detailed manual describing the scoring criteria is available (Marengo, Harrow et al., in press). Inter-rater reliability ranged from .67 to .91 for the three tests. This composite measure of bizarre-idiosyncratic thinking has been used successfully in previous research on positive thought disorder (Harrow, Silverstein

Table 6.3
Prevalence of Negative Symptoms, Intellectual Deficit, and Positive Symptoms in Chronic Schizophrenia

Negative Symptoms				
	Poverty of Speech	Flat Affect	Psychomotor Retardation	Total Score
M (SD)	1.41 (1.93)	1.19 (1.97)	0.46 (0.95)	3.06 (3.99)
N (%)*	4 (26%)	16 (30%)	5 (9%)	17 (32%
Intellectual Deficit				
	Information	Comprehension	Digit Symbol Substitution Test (DSST)	
M (SD)†	7.17 (3.51)	6.13 (3.55)	5.88 (3.58)	
N (%)‡	24 (44%)	31 (57%)	37 (72%)	
Positive Symptoms				
	Hallucinations	Delusions	Positive Thought Disorder	Overall Positive Symptom Index
N (%)§	21 (44%)	29 (59%)	34 (63%)	47 (87%)

Note: Percentages adjusted for missing data.

* Patients with a score of 2 or greater on individual negative symptom scales, or 4 or greater on the total score.

† Age-standardized scale scores (Wechsler, 1955).

‡ Patients one standard deviation below the mean of Wechsler's (1955) standardization sample (age-corrected score less than 7).

§ Patients with definite ratings of positive symptoms.

et al., 1983; Marengo & Harrow, in press). As a parallel to the negative symptom Total Score, an Overall Positive Symptom Index (Pogue-Geile & Harrow, 1984a) was developed based on the presence of any one of the following: hallucinations, delusions, or the composite measure of bizarre-idiosyncratic thinking. This Overall Positive Symptom Index was scaled as: 1) positive symptoms absent; 2) at least one mild or equivocal, but no definite ratings; and 3) at least one definite rating.

RESULTS

Prevalence of Negative Symptoms, Intellectual Deficit, and Positive Symptoms

Table 6.3 presents the prevalence of negative symptoms, intellectual deficit and positive symptoms in this hospitalized, chronic schizophrenic sample. Flat affect was the most frequent of the negative symptoms, with 30 percent of the schizophrenics showing this sign to a marked degree. Poverty of speech was almost as common (26%), and psychomotor retardation was the least frequent (9%) negative symptom in this sample. Overall, 32 percent of the patients evidenced definite behavioral signs of a negative symptom syndrome. Thus, overt negative symptoms occurred in only a minority of these severely disordered, chronic schizophrenics.

The extent of intellectual deficit in this sample was quite marked. In terms of age-standardized scores (mean = 10 and standard deviation = 3 in a normal population), the means in this group for all three tests of intellectual functioning were well below the norm. The DSST test of psychomotor speed showed the lowest performance, followed by the Comprehension test and the Information test. Fully 72 percent of these chronic schizophrenics performed one standard deviation below the mean of the normal population on psychomotor speed and 44 percent fell one standard deviation below the norm on the test of general information. Whether a function of low premorbid intellectual levels or deterioration, it is clear that substantial intellectual deficit, particularly in psychomotor speed, was present in a large subgroup of these chronic schizophrenics.

Table 6.3 also presents the prevalence of positive symptoms. Positive symptoms were quite frequent. Severe positive thought disorder and delusions were the most common positive symptoms. Overall, 87 percent of these chronic schizophrenics showed at least one definite positive symptom at the time of testing. In one view, the severe level of positive symptoms might be expected since all the patients had met the criteria for schizophrenia according to the NHSI at admission for their current hospitalization. However, a number of recent theorists have proposed that positive symptoms should be less important in the later phases of chronic schizophrenia. The present results do not support this latter view.

Demographic and Clinical Correlates of Negative Symptoms and Intellectual Deficit

There were no significant associations between negative symptoms and the standard demographic variables of current age, sex, or age at first hospitalization. In contrast, the duration of the disorder, as indexed by the number of years since first hospitalization, was significantly associated in a positive direction with the presence of negative symptoms (Total Score) ($r=.27$, $p < .05$). There was also a nonsignificant trend for lifetime total duration of hospitalization to be related in a positive direction to negative symptoms (Total Score) ($r=.24$, $p < .05$). Therefore, the subgroup of schizophrenics with negative symptoms tended to have been ill longer and to have spent somewhat more time hospitalized than those without negative symptoms.

There were no significant associations between any of the three indices of intellectual functioning and the demographic variables of sex, age, or number of previous hospitalizations. However, low performances on Information and Comprehension tests were significantly associated with a longer duration of disorder (years since first hospitalization) (Information, $r = -.35$, $p < .01$; Comprehension, $r = -.40$, $p < .004$) and with increased time spent hospitalized (Information, $r = -.42$, $p < .002$; Comprehension, $r = -.41$, $p < .002$). In contrast, deficits on the DSST were only significantly associated with an early age of first hospitalization ($r = .36$, $p < .012$). The Information and Comprehension tests were not significantly associated with age of onset. In summary, patients with severe deficits in knowledge and social comprehension tended to have been ill longer and to have spent more time hospitalized. This is a similar pattern to that shown by the behavioral negative symptoms. Psychomotor retardation differed from this pattern.

Relationship Between Negative Symptoms and Intellectual Functioning

Table 6.4 presents the association between negative symptoms and the three measures of intellectual functioning. These associations were strongest for poverty of speech and flat affect and did not differ significantly between males and females. These results suggest that these two classes of deficit may be influenced by some common factor.

In contrast, negative symptoms were only modestly associated with the patients' amount of education, although the relationship between flat affect and education was significant. This suggests that early educational failure only increased slightly the later risk for

Table 6.4
Association Between Negative Symptoms and Intellectual Functioning in Chronic Schizophrenics†

	Intellectual Functioning			
	Information Test	Compre-hension Test	Digit Symbol Substitution Test	Education
Negative Symptom				
Poverty of Speech	-.29**	-.34***	.36***	-.11
Flat Affect	-.24**	-.21**	-.19*	-.15*
Psychomotor Retardation	-.18*	-.17*	-.11	-.04
Total Score	-.31***	-.33***	-.32***	-.14
Education	.30**	.18*	.22*	
Positive Symptom				
Hallucinations	-.10	.04	-.07	-.07
Delusions	.02	.04	.16	-.10
Positive Thought Disorder	-.30**	-.27**	-.08	-.03
Overall Positive Symptom Index	-.02	.06	.08	.02

† Kendall's Tau C, N = 54
* $p < .05$
** $p < .01$
*** $p < .001$

negative symptoms in these chronic schizophrenics. In more acute, younger samples, we have found that educational failure is more strongly associated with the development of negative symptoms (Pogue-Geile & Harrow, 1984a). As would be expected, intellectual functioning was also significantly related to educational level, as is presented in Table 6.4.

Partial correlational analyses were performed to explore the role that educational attainment might play in the relationship between negative symptoms and current intellectual functioning. Significant correlations between current intellectual functioning and negative symptoms remained after partialling-out the variation in level of education (Negative Symptom Total Score with Information,

$r = .35$, $p < .01$; Comprehension $r = .42$, p .002; DSST, $r=-.34$, $p < .01$ controlling for educational level). This result suggests that the covariation in negative symptoms and intellectual functioning in this older, chronic sample may be due to more recent factors than earlier educational achievement or factors that influenced educational level.

Relationship Between Positive Symptoms and Intellectual Functioning

Table 6.4 also presents the relationship between positive symptoms and intellectual functioning. In general, two positive symptoms (hallucinations and delusions) were not significantly associated with these measures of intellectual performance either in the total group or in males and females separately. The third positive symptom, positive thought disorder, correlated significantly with the Information and Comprehension tests, such that thought disorder was associated with poor intellectual performance. It is likely that thought disorder or factors underlying it (e.g., disorganization) may interfere with verbal performance on these tests since even our measures of thought disorder that are not based on the Comprehension test were significantly correlated with the intellectual tests. Table 6.4 also shows the absence of any significant relationship between educational level and positive symptoms.

Relationship Between Negative and Positive Symptoms

Table 6.5 presents the relationship between negative and positive symptoms. Only one of these associations was significant, and the rest were quite low. This pattern also occurred in both males and females separately. These data suggest that even within chronic schizophrenia, positive and negative symptoms are not at opposite ends of a bipolar dimension, but rather that in the present situation they tend to be independent of each other. Thus, it would appear that the processes immediately underlying these classes of symptoms are not mutually exclusive or antagonistic.

Relevant to the same issue, the lower half of Table 6.5 presents a categorical analysis of the relationship between positive and negative symptoms. This analysis also demonstrates the independence of positive and negative symptoms in this sample. The most frequent profile was that of schizophrenics with only positive symptoms and without definite negative symptoms (59%). Next most frequent was a mixed profile with both definite positive and definite negative symptoms (28%). A pure negative symptom type, without positive symptoms, was quite rare (4%) in this chronic population. These data present further evidence that even in this severely

Table 6.5
Association Between Negative and Positive Symptoms in Chronic Schizophrenics

	Negative Symptom*			
Positive Symptom	Poverty of Speech	Flat Affect	Psychomotor Retrardation	Total Score
Hallucinations	.13	- .02	.19†	.04
Delusions	.03	.03	.09	- .02
Positive Thought Disorder	.02	- .03	.01	.00
Overall Positive Symptom Index	- .04	- .04	.06	- .06

	Categorical Analysis‡			
Overall Positive Symptom Index	Overall Negative Symptom Index			
	Absent/Mild		Definite	
Absent/Mild	5	(9%)	2	(4%)
Definite	32	(59%)	15	(28%)

* Kendall's Tau C, N = 54.

† $p < .05$

‡ N = 54. $X^2 = .03$, $p = .86$.

disturbed group of schizophrenics positive and negative symptoms are not mutually exclusive.

Joint Negative/Positive Subgroups and Intellectual Functioning

Some theorists have proposed categorizing patients on the basis of their joint negative/positive symptom profile (e.g., Andreasen, & Olsen 1982). In order to explore this approach in relation to intellectual functioning, patients were classified into four subgroups based on the presence of definite negative and/or positive symptoms: 1) negative only, 2) mixed positive and negative, 3) positive only, and 4) neither symptom to a definite degree. Table 6.6 presents the mean scores on intellectual functioning for these four groups. Although sample sizes in some of the groups were small, separate 2-way ANOVAs (Negative symptoms x Positive symptoms) for each of the measures of intellectual functioning produced similar results. Significant main effects were found for the negative symptom factor for all three measures (Information, $F = 7.15$, $p < .01$; Comprehension,

Table 6.6
Relationship Between Joint Negative/Positive Subgroups and Intellectual Functioning

	Joint Negative/Positive Subgroup			
Intellectual Funtioning	Negative Only (N = 2)	Mixed Positive & Negative (N = 15)	Positive Only (N = 32)	Neither Symptom (N = 5)
Information	6.50	5.40	8.17	8.20
Comprehension	3.50	4.27	7.66	5.60
Digit Symbol Substitution Test	3.50	4.60	6.62	6.40

Note: Means. Age-standardized, higher scores denote better performance.

$F=11.65$, $p < .001$; DSST, $F=4.12$, $p < .05$). In contrast, the main effects for positive symptoms and the interactions of negative and positive symptoms were not significant. These results suggest, consistent with analyses presented above, that only negative symptoms were associated with intellectual deficit. In addition, this association seems to be relatively unaffected by the presence or absence of positive symptoms in this sample of chronic schizophrenics.

DISCUSSION

To summarize, the present research sought to investigate within a chronic schizophrenic population some of the primary hypotheses concerning negative symptoms. The following major results emerged;

1) Negative symptoms were present in a subgroup but not all of these hospitalized chronic schizophrenics.
2) Substantial intellectual deficits characterized many of these hospitalized chronic schizophrenics.
3) Negative symptoms were significantly associated with intellectual deficits.
4) Positive symptoms were present in a large percentage of these chronic schizophrenics, in contrast with some current hypotheses.
5) Hallucinations and delusions, two major positive symptoms, were not associated with intellectual

deficits, whereas positive thought disorder was related to intellectual deficits.

6) Negative and positive symptoms were not intercorrelated and were not at opposite ends of a bipolar dimension.
7) The relationship between negative symptoms and intellectual deficit was not modified by the presence of positive symptoms.

Considering that these chronic schizophrenics may be thought of as at "high risk" for negative symptoms, it is important that only a subgroup of them showed negative symptoms. Other studies have also found marked negative symptoms to occur primarily in a subgroup of chronic schizophrenics rather than in all of them (Johnstone, Crow et al., 1978; Opler, Kay, et al., 1984; Owens & Johnstone, 1980. In addition, other studies of young, acute inpatients (Andreasen, 1979b; Andreasen & Olsen, 1982), and young patients at follow-up one year after hospital discharge (Pogue-Geile & Harrow, 1984a; 1984b) also report that definite negative symptoms occur in only a minority of schizophrenics. These findings suggest that it is likely that marked negative symptoms are relevant to only a subgroup of schizophrenics, as they are currently defined, rather than to all schizophrenics.

Another striking finding of this study was the extent of intellectual deficit present in these chronic patients. Similar results with other measures of cognitive impairment have been reported in other studies of chronic schizophrenic inpatients (e.g., Heaton, Baade et al., 1978; Liddle & Crow, 1984; Owens & Johnstone, 1980; Stevens, Crow et al., 1978). Although it is difficult to use these findings to estimate the precise prevalence of intellectual dysfunction in schizophrenia in general, it is clear that severe cognitive deficits do occur in a definite subgroup of schizophrenics at sometime during the course of their disorder.

Our results also suggest that negative symptoms mark a subgroup of these chronic schizophrenics who show particularly poor cognitive functioning across a variety of tests. Other studies are consistent with this finding in older, chronic schizophrenics (Lilliston 1973; Depue, 1976; Johnstone, Crow et al., 1978; Owens & Johnstone, 1980; Johnstone, Owens et al., 1981), although it is unclear how strong this association is in younger patients. Our preliminary analyses of young, acute schizophrenics at follow-up find somewhat weaker associations between negative symptoms and intellectual functioning.

The exact nature of this association between intellectual functioning and negative symptoms in the present data is such that most schizophrenics with negative symptoms show intellectual deficit, but many schizophrenics experience intellectual deficit without marked negative symptoms. For example, 94% of schizophrenics with definite negative symptoms had scores on the Information test one standard deviation or more below the norm, but 61% of patients with such intellectual deficits did not show definite signs of negative symptoms at the time. These data may indicate that a common factor may influence both negative symptoms and intellectual deficit in some schizophrenics, but that intellectual deficit may be heterogeneous in this population. These findings also support the heuristic value of the notion that we proposed earlier, that cognitive deficits can also be considered a kind of negative symptom, along with the traditional behavioral deficit syndromes of poverty of speech and flat affect. Pogue-Geile and Harrow (1984a) have proposed that these traditional negative symptoms be termed Type A negative symptoms and that cognitive deficits be classified as Type B negative symptoms.

These results are generally consistent with Crow's hypothesis (1980) that some structural brain abnormality, such as cortical atrophy, may underlie both negative symptoms and intellectual deficit in some schizophrenics, although we do not have CT scan data for these patients. The number of studies that have found ventricular enlargement on CT scan to be associated with cognitive impairment (Type B negative symptoms) in schizophrenia provide stronger tests of this hypothesis (Johnstone, Crow et al., 1976; Johnstone, Crow et al., 1978; Rieder, Donnelly et al., 1979; Donnelly, Wienberger et al., 1980; Golden, Moses et al., 1980; Golden, Macinnes et al., 1982). However, despite initial suggestive reports (Johnstone, Crow et al., 1976) recent studies have failed to find significant associations between ventricular enlargement on CT scan and negative behavioral symptoms (Type A negative symptoms) (Andreasen, Olsen et al., 1982; Nasrallah, Kuperman et al., 1983; Luchins, Lewine et al., 1984). These inter- relationships among ventricular enlargement, negative symptoms, and cognitive deficit require further study, but the findings to date may suggest a more complex picture than that originally hypothesized by Crow (1980) in which some structural brain abnormality would produce both intellectual deficit and negative behavioral symptoms. For example, it may be that cognitive deficits (Type B negative symptoms) may provide a better indicator than Type A behavioral negative symptoms of structural brain abnormalities. Thus, although our results are consistent with Crow's hypothesis, they do not provide a strong test of its biological aspects, and are compatible with alternative hypotheses. For example, it may be that low premorbid intellectual ability (due to independent factors) serves as a risk factor for negative symptoms if a person later becomes schizophrenic. However, the finding that many schizophrenics evidence intellectual deficit without showing negative symptoms would argue that cognitive deficits alone are not sufficient to lead to negative symptoms in schizophrenia.

Our results on the relationship between negative and positive symptoms in chronic schizophrenia also have important implications for theory. The data indicate that negative and positive symptoms do not tend to be mutually exclusive or negatively correlated. Other studies with young schizophrenics at follow-up (Pogue-Geile & Harrow, 1983a, 1984a), young inpatients (Lewine, Fogg et al., 1983), and older, chronic schizophrenics (Johnstone, Owens et al., 1981; reanalysis of Opler, Kay et al., 1984) have all reported the absence of any inverse relationship between negative and positive symptoms (cf. Andreasen & Olsen, 1982). This implies that the processes immediately underlying these two classes of symptoms are not antagonistic. In addition, the fact that negative symptoms occur in a substantial subgroup of schizophrenics (Pogue-Geile & Harrow, 1984a), all of whom at one time had experienced positive symptoms, further suggests that the processes underlying these two classes of symptoms must in fact be *positively* associated in some longitudinal manner. This is particularly true if one considers the larger population of all psychiatric patients, where negative symptoms are most common in schizophrenics and to some degree other psychotic patients, and less frequent in non-psychotic groups (Pogue-Geile & Harrow, 1984b). Such findings argue strongly for a positive association between negative and positive symptoms in this larger population.

Conjectures on Potential Etiologies of Negative Symptoms

While Crow (1980) has proposed several stimulating hypotheses concerning the possible organic pathology of negative symptoms, less discussion has centered on the potential etiology of negative symptoms. Although there are few studies specifically relevant to this issue, the evidence to date appears to indicate that negative symptoms have enough important correlates that some attention to the etiological possibilities is warranted. Since severe negative symptoms are probably only relevant to a subgroup of schizophrenics, as they are currently diagnosed, we will outline three general models that would be applicable to individual differences within schizophrenia such as negative symptoms.

First, in a "modifying influence" model, negative symptoms would develop as the result of an interaction between some independent trait, such as low intelligence, and the more specific schizophrenic (or psychotic) diathesis. In this case, the independent trait does not actually increase the risk for schizophrenia itself, but only serves to modulate the phenotypic manifestation of schizophrenia. The etiology of the independent trait itself could be genetic and/or environmental. In the case of such a modifying influence etiology, negative symptoms, although identifying a *subgroup* of schizophrenics, would not generally be considered to have identified a *subtype* of schizophenia with some specific etiology.

A second etiological possibility is a "contributing influence" model in which negative symptoms represent the behavioral manifestation of some "negative symptom specific" factor that not only leads to negative symptoms, but also directly contributes to the risk of schizophrenia. This negative symptom specific factor could itself be due to genetic and/or environmental influences. For example, within the context of a polygenic theory of schizophrenia in which three of five "schizophrenia specific" genes (A, B, C, D, E) are necessary to produce clinical schizophrenia, then any schizophrenic who has the "negative symptom" gene ('D') as one of his three genes will show negative symptoms. In the extreme case where the 'D' gene is sufficient to produce a schizophrenic picture, then negative symptom schizophrenia would represent a distinct type of schizophrenia with its own specific etiology. A similar example could be fashioned for a putative environmental factor, such as viral infection which could both lead to negative symptoms and also contribute to the risk of schizophrenia.

In the third, or "threshold model," negative symptoms would represent a behavioral marker of a more severe threshold along a continuum of multifactorial liability to schizophrenia. In this case, negative symptoms would not be due to any specific influence, but would reflect only the number of negative symptom-nonspecific influences present for any given individual. Within the context of the polygenic example give above, where three schizophrenia-specific genes are necessary to produce clinical schizophrenia, it could be that four of the five genes would be necessary to produce schizophrenia with negative symptoms (the negative symptoms threshold). In this case no one of the five genes would be specific for negative symptoms, but only the total number of genes present would be important.

This range of potential models for the etiology of negative symptoms does not exhaust all the possibilities and although they are quite general, they can provide a framework for investigating these issues and are specific enough to make different predictions in the context of family and twin studies. These models also have been discussed in reference to the traditional subtypes of schizophrenia (e.g., Gottesman & Shields, 1982). Although much more needs to be understood concerning the behavioral and biological correlates of negative symptoms, studies of etiological questions may provide new insights into the role that negative symptoms might play in schizophrenia and other disorders.

REFERENCES

Andreasen, N.C. (1979a). Thought, language, and communication disorders: II. Diagnostic significance. *Arch. Gen. Psychiatry*, 36:1325-1330.

Andreasen, N.C. (1979b). Affective flattening and the criteria for schizophrenia. *Am. J. Psychiatry*, 136:944-947.

Andreasen, N.C. (1981). *Scale for the Assessment of Negative Symptoms (SANS)*. Iowa City, Iowa: The University of Iowa.

Andreasen, N.C. (1982). Negative symptoms in schizophrenia: Definition and reliability. *Arch. Gen. Psychiatry*, 39:784-788.

Andreasen, N.C. and Olsen, S. (1982). Negative versus positive schizophrenia: Definition and validation. *Arch. Gen. Psychiatry*, 39:789-794.

Andreasen, N.C., Olsen, S.A., Dennert, J.W., and Smith, M.R. (1982). Ventricular enlargement in schizophrenia: Relationships to positive and negative schizophrenia. *Am. J. Psychiatry*, 139:297-302.

Astrachan, B.M., Harrow, M., Adler, D., Schwartz, A., Schwartz, C., and Tucker, G. (1972). A checklist for the diagnosis of schizophrenia. *Brit. J. Psychiatry*, 121:529-539.

Bleuler, E. (1950). *Dementia Praecox or the Group of Schizophrenias*. Translated by J. Zinkin. New York: International Universities Press.

Bridge, T.P., Cannon, H.E., and Wyatt, R.J. (1978). Burned-out schizophrenia: Evidence for age effects on schizophrenic symptomatology. *J. Gerontology*, 33:835-839.

Carpenter, W.T., Sacks, M.H., Strauss, J.S., Bartko, J.J., and Rayner, J. (1976). Evaluating signs and symptoms: Comparisons of structured interview and clinical approaches. *Brit. J. Psychiatry*, 128:397-403.

Chapman, C.J. and Chapman, J.P. (1973). *Disordered Thought in Schizophrenia*. Englewood, Cliffs, NJ: Prentice Hall, Inc.

Crow, T.J. (1980). Molecular pathology of schizophrenia: More than one disease process? *Brit. Med. J.*, 280:1-9.

Crow, T.J. (1982). The biology of schizophrenia. *Experientia*, 38:1275-1282.

Depue, R.A. (1975). An activity-withdrawal distinction in schizophrenia: Behavioral, clinical, brain damage, and neuropsychological correlates. *J. Abnl. Psychology*, 85:174-185.

Donnelly, E.F., Weinberger, D.R., Waldman, I.N., and Wyatt, R.J. (1980). Cognitive impairment associated with morphological brain abnormalities on computed tomography in chronic schizophrenic patients. *J. Nerv. Ment. Dis.*, 168:305-308.

Fish, F.J. (1962). *Schizophrenia*. Baltimore: Williams & Wilkins Co.

Golden, C.J., Macinnes, W.D., Ariel, R.N., Ruedrich, S.L., Chu, C., Coffman, J.A., Graber, B., and Bloch, S. (1982). Cross-validation of the ability of the Luria-Nebraska Neuropsychological Battery to differentiate chronic schizophrenics with and without ventricular enlargement. *J. Consult. Clin. Psychology*, 50:87-95.

Golden, C.J., Moses, J.A., Zelazowski, R., Graber, B., Zatz, L.M., Horvath, T.B., and Berger, P.A. (1980). Cerebral ventricular size and neuropsychological impairment in young chronic schizophrenics. *Arch. Gen. Psychiatry*, 37:610-623.

Goldstein, K. and Scheerer, M. (1941). Abstract and concrete behavior: An experimental study with special tests. *Psychological Monographs*, 1941, 53, Whole No. 2.

Gorham, D. Use of the proverbs test for differentiating schizophrenics from normals. *J. Consult. Clin. Psychology*, 20:434-440.

Gottesman, I.I. and Shields, J. (1982). *Schizophrenia: The Epigenetic Puzzle*. New York: Cambridge University Press.

Grinker, R.R., Sr. and Harrow, M. (Eds.). (in press). *A Multidimensional Approach to Clinical Research in Schizophrenia*. Springfield, Ill: Charles C Thomas.

Harrow, M., Marengo, J., Pogue-Geile, M.F., and Pawelski, T.J. (in press). Schizophrenic deficits in intelligence and abstract thinking: Influence of aging and long-term institutionalization. In N. Miller (Ed.). (in press). *Schizophrenia, Paranoia, and Schizophreniform Disorders in Later Life*. New York: Guilford Press.

Harrow, M. and Quinlan, D. (in press). *Disordered Thinking and Schizophrenic Psychopathology*. New York: Gardner Press.

Harrow, M., Silverstein, M., and Marengo, J. (1983). Disordered thinking: Does it identify nuclear schizophrenia? *Arch. Gen Psychiatry*, 40:765-771.

Heaton, R.K., Baade, L.E., and Johnson, K.L. (1978). Neuropsychological test results associated with psychiatric disorders in adults. *Psychological Bulletin*, 85:141-162.

Huber, G., Gross, G., Schuttler, R., and Linz, M. (1980). Longitudinal studies of schizophrenic patients. *Schizophrenia Bulletin*, 6:592-605.

Jackson, J.H. (1887). Remarks on evolution and dissolution of the nervous system. *J. Ment. Science*, 33:25-48.

Johnstone, E.C., Crow, T.J., Frith, C.D., Husband, J., and Kreel, L. (1976). Cerebral ventricular size and cognitive impairment in chronic schizophrenia. *Lancet*, 2:924-926.

Johnstone, E.C., Crow, T.J., Frith, C.D., Stevens, M., Kreel, L., and Husband, J. (1978). The dementia of dementia praecox. *Acta Psychiatrica Scandinavica*, 56:305-324

Johnstone, E.C., Owens, D.G.C., Gold, A., Crow, T.J., and MacMillan, J.F. (1981). Institutionalization and the defects of schizophrenia. *Brit. J. Psychiatry*, 139:195-203.

Kraepelin, E. (1919). *Dementia Praecox*. Translated by R.M. Barclay. Edinburgh: E.S. Livingstone Ltd.

Lewine, R.R.J., Fogg, L., and Meltzer, H.Y. (1983). Assessment of negative and positive symptoms in schizophrenia. *Schizophrenia Bulletin*, 9:368-376.

Liddle, P.F. and Crow, T.J. (1984). Age disorientation in chronic schizophrenia is associated with global intellectual impairment. *Brit. J. Psychiatry*, 144:193-199.

Lilliston, L. (1973). Schizophrenic symptomatology as a function of probability of cerebral damage. *J. Abnl. Psychology*, 82:377-381.

Luchins, D.J., Lewine, R.R.J., and Meltzer, H.Y. (1984). Lateral ventricular size, psychopathology, and medication response in the psychoses. *Biological Psychiatry*, 19:29- 44.

Marengo, J. and Harrow, M. (in press). Thought disorder: A function of schizophrenia, mania, or psychosis? *J. Nerv. Ment. Dis.*

Marengo, J., Harrow, M., Lanin, I., and Wilson, A. (in press). A manual for assessing aspects of bizarre-idiosyncratic thinking. In M. Harrow and D. Quinlan (Eds.), *Disordered Thinking and Schizophrenic Psychopathology*. New York: Gardner Press.

Nasrallah, H.A., Kuperman, S., Hamra, B.J., and McCalley-Whitters, M. (1983). Clinical differences between schizophrenic patients with and without large cerebral ventricles. *J. Clin. Psychiatry*, 44:407-409.

Opler, L.A., Kay, S.R., Rosado, V., and Lindenmayer, J. (1984). Positive and negative syndromes in chronic schizophrenic inpatients. *J. Nerv. Ment. Dis.*, 172:317-325.

Owens, D.G.C. and Johnstone, E.C. (1980). The disabilities of chronic schizophrenia: Their nature and the factors contributing to their development. *Brit. J. Psychiatry*, 136:384-395.

Pogue-Geile, M.F. and Harrow, M. (1983a). Are negative symptoms specific to schizophrenia? *Scientific Proceedings of the American Psychiatric Association*, 275. Washington, D.C.: American Psychiatric Association.

Pogue-Geile, M.F. and Harrow, M. (1983b). *The Longitudinal Study of Negative Symptoms in Schizophrenia: Psychomotor Retardation.* Presented at the 91st Annual Meeting of the American Psychological Association.

Pogue-Geile, M.F. and Harrow, M. (1984a). Negative and positive symptoms in schizophrenia and depression: A follow-up study. *Schizophrenia Bulletin*, 10:371-387.

Pogue-Geile, M.F. and Harrow, M. (1984b). *Negative Symptoms in Schizophrenia and Other Psychoses.* Presented at the 92nd Annual Meeting of the American Psychological Association.

Pogue-Geile, M.F., Harrow, M., and Marengo, J. (1983). *Negative Symptoms and Intellectual Deficit in Chronic Schizophrenia.* Presented at the 55th Annual Meeting of the Midwestern Psychological Association.

Pogue-Geile, M.F., Harrow, M., and Marengo, J. (1984). The prognosis of schizophrenic negative symptoms. *Scientific Proceedings of the American Psychiatric Association*, 256. Washington, D.C., American Psychiatric Association.

Reynolds, H.T. (1977). *The Analysis of Cross-Classifications.* New York: The Free Press.

Rieder, R.D., Donnelly, E.F., Herdt, F.R., and Waldman, I.N. (1979). Sulcal prominence in young chronic schizophrenic patients: CT scan findings associated with impairment on neuropsychological tests. *Psychiatry Research*, 1:1-8.

Rubin, N.S., Pogue-Geile, M.F., Harrow, M., and Cohler, B. (1983). *Positive and Negative Symptoms in the Early Course of Schizophrenia.* Presented at the 91st Annual Meeting of the American Psychological Association.

Spitzer, R.L. and Endicott, J. (1978). *Schedule for Affective Disorders and Schizophrenia* (SADS). New York, N.Y.: Biometrics Research, New York State Psychiatric Institute.

Stevens, M., Crow, T.J., Bowman, M.J., and Coles, E.C. (1978). Age disorientation in schizophrenia: A constant prevalence of 25 percent in a chronic mental hospital population. *Brit. J. Psychiatry*, 133:130-136.

Strauss, J.S. and Carpenter, W.T. (1974). *The Psychiatric Assessment Interview* (PAI). New Haven, Ct.: Yale University.

Strauss, J.S., Carpenter, W.T., and Bartko, J.J. (1974). Speculations on the processes that underlie schizophrenic symptoms and signs. *Schizophrenia Bulletin*, 11:61-69.

Wechsler, D. (1955). *Wechsler Adult Intelligence Scale Manual*. New York: Psychological Corporation.

Wing, J.K. (1978). Clinical concepts of schizophrenia. In J.K. Wing (Ed.), *Schizophrenia: Towards a New Synthesis*. New York: Grune & Stratton.

Wing, J.K. and Brown, G.W. (1970). *Institutionalism and Schizophrenia*. London: Cambridge University Press.

World Health Organization. (1973). *The International Pilot Study of Schizophrenia*. Geneva: World Health Organization.

7

The Hedonic Element in Affectivity

*HENRY KRYSTAL**

The hedonic quality of affects is, commonly prevailing impression to the contrary, not an inherent, inseparable part of the emotions. A study of conditions in which there are changes in the subjective quality of emotions, such as anhedonia, or the so-called "libidinization" of affects, indicates that the quality of pleasure and distress is separate, and is only epigenetically linked with the rest of the complex experience which constitutes emotions. A metaphoric view of the anatomic and physiological apparatus illustrates this conception and further suggests that in infancy, before affects are matured enough to be utilizable as signals, the direct experience and distress provides the qualitative signal. This response becomes an essential factor in self- and object- representation formation.

The assumption is commonly made that some emotions are intrinsically and invariably pleasurable and others equally constantly unpleasant or painful. I question this assumption, particularly because it does not square with certain clinical syndromes in which the hedonic quality of affects changes. I propose that the adult experience of affects is a blend of self-perception of responses from several sources. Among the elements of the emotion are the perceptions of pleasure or distress, which derive from a phylogenetically and ontogenetically ancient somatic and mental apparatus. The experiences of pleasure or distress become quite closely related to certain emotions, but their separate derivation makes possible later shifts in quality of pleasure in affects. The understanding of these shifts is necessary in order to deal with anhedonia, as well as such phenomena as "libidinization" of anxiety and other affects. Rather

* This is a modified version of a paper which was originally published in the Annual of Psychoanalysis 9:93-114, 1981. I wish to thank Dr. G. Pollock, Chairman, Editorial Board, The Chicago Institute for Psychoanalysis and the International Universities Press, for their kind permission to use this material.

than thinking of emotions as unitary phenomena, it is helpful to consider their identifiable elements.

CONCEPTIONS OF AFFECTS

I will not attempt a complete review of the history of the ways in which emotions have been described and conceptualized. Freud's view of emotions, which is the one most familiar to psychoanalysis, simply reflected the physiological and psychiatric attitudes of his age. It was burdened with the mind-body schism, and with a mechanistic attitude toward the body processes. The tendency to think of mental function as a reflex arc produced an inclination to consider emotions as discharge phenomena. Freud saw the bond between the cognitive and expressive aspects of emotions as a fairly loose one. The feebleness of the bonding between ideas and emotions permitted ego defenses such as a reversal, displacement, or complete suppression of affects (Freud, 1926). Freud's absorption with the idea that emotions were discharge phenomena made it impossible for him to consider emotions as unconscious, even when he found clinical evidence of such forces as the unconscious sense of guilt (1907, 1923). With his recognition of signal anxiety (1926) he did give us a way to conceptualize affects as related to ego function, but never quite got around to adjusting the view of emotions accordingly. In my earlier writings (Krystal and Raskin, 1970) I have reviewed the evidence that signal affects are essential to such functions as perception, cognition, memory, and recall. Through these many subliminal functions, signal affects provide protection against traumatization.

It appears that affects are utilizable as signals only after having undergone the maturational processes of differentiation, desomatization, and verbalization (Krystal, 1970; 1974). However, a consideration of the above sequence reveals a serious theoretical problem concealed in it. If we postulate that the utilizability of affects as signals depends upon their having undergone a processes of differentiation and verbalization-desomatization, we would expect that with affect regression there would be a serious impairment in virtually all ego functions – certainly in those which have been demonstrated to involve signal affects. *Moreover, the expectation that the maturation of affects would have to precede the development of such basic functions as perception seems to be in conflict with the basic assumptions of object-relations, and self- and object-representation in early life.*

We have, of course, no way of knowing how perceptions are processed in the infant and how they are registered, or when they start leaving lasting memories. But it is startling and puzzling to consider that there are some adults whose affects have undergone imperfect development or regression, and who consequently have difficulties in utilizing their emotions as signals to themselves. These individuals show a disturbance in object-relations, a lack of empathy with the significant objects in their lives, and even a tendency to treat themselves as robots. If that is so, then we could assume that in the young child, in whom the affects have not yet reached maturity, the perception and registration of object-representations has to be different than the kind we discover in the best functioning adults. And yet, in psychoanalytic theory, we have assumed that individuals keep forming object representations of some kind from the beginning – even before a recognition of the separatness of the self-representation from the object-representation is effected. Moreover, the assumption was always made that emotions were involved in these object-representations. For instance, Kernberg (1976) stated: "My formulations imply that cathexes are, first of all, affective cathexes, that is, the quantitative element or economic factor involved in the intensity of primitive affect dispositions, which are activated in the context of primitive units of internalized object relations and constitute the organizers of such primitive units" (p. 113). He further stresses: "Cathexes are first of all affect cathexis" (p. 114). The same author has elaborated the point in 1982:

> Affects, operating as the earliest motivational system, are therefore intimately linked with the fixation by memory of internalized object relations. I would suggest that affects are the primary motivational system in the sense that they are at the center of each of the infinite number of gratifying and frustrating concrete events the infant experiences with his environment. Affects link a series of undifferentiated self-object representations so that gradually a complex world of internalized object relations, some pleasurably tinged, others unpleasurably tinged is constructed. (p. 907).

With the renewal of interest in the process of attachment (Bowlby, 1969) and the studies on attachment behavior (Ainsworth, Blehar, Walter and Wall, 1978; Parkes and Stevenson-Hinde, 1982) the schedule of attachment has been moved back to as early as two to seven months of age (Greenspan, 1981). We must wonder: in these early stages of development what could be the nature of the affect signals on the capacity to register them?

Bowlby (1969) assumed "affects and emotions" to be available from the start as appraising processes. Bowlby later (1973) made explicit his view that in all the attachment steps, including its earliest precursors, the affects of security, fear, anxiety and anger were indispensible tools of the whole process. Biologically oriented students of depression find the most reliable way to produce an animal model of it is by separating the young from their mother (J.H. Krystal, 1984). If the mother is not quickly restored and the child survives, serious impairment of all affective development and of all ego functions will ensue. But let us ask now: how can it be that primal self and object representations can develop at an early time, before any affect signals have yet evolved through desomatization and differentiation? And how do these object relations develop at all, if there is no affect *signal* available in a form suitable for the development of a "loving memory"? We have postulated an interdependence in these processes without having provision for one of them to mature enough to be available for the other. What is the way out of this dilemma? Have we arrived at another "non-liquet?"

A possible solution offers itself in the consideration of the distress or psychic pain signal as separately derived from the rest of the affect experience. However, before we can explore it, we must critically examine our conceptions of the emotions to see if such a possibility is feasible.

The need to reconsider psychoanalytic conceptions of affect arises from other difficulties as well. One of these problems derives from the "discharge" theory of affect, which represents an uncritical incorporation of the common idea that the affects are sporadic, occasional occurrences (Krystal, 1978b). Current views of affect are much more in harmony with Cannon's (1927) idea that every perception and every mental event is accompanied by an "emotional quota." He acknowledged that the affective component was not always conscious and tried to account for it by a theory that affects were primarily thalamically registered and only became conscious if cortical inhibition was abolished. In the long view of theories and conceptions of affects, the "discharge" formulation is by no means the only or even the predominant one. In fact, it is amazing how many interpretations and theories of affects have been advanced. In the multiplicity of hypotheses about the nature of emotions I have found one that describes them as having "three dimensions" which I hope to demonstrate have disparate psychological and physiological bases. Wundt (1920) suggested that the three dimensions of feeling were: (1) pleasantness (unpleasantness), (2) tension (relaxation), and (3) excitement (quiescence). The question is whether these elements in the subjective experience of affects are indeed intrinsic, inseparable parts of a given affect.

Offhand, one is inclined to assert that certain emotions are always pleasant, others distressing, and that each emotion has a characteristic level of arousal. But, upon reflection, one discovers that, even in the normal individual, emotions vary considerably in the degree of pleasure or unpleasure. Even anxiety may be quite pleasurable, and in fact is a regular source of "thrills." Anxiety and variety (in the sense of divergence between a perception and the accustomed expectation) are the most effective "arousers" (Pribram, 1968).

THE TERMS: LIBIDINIZATION, SEXUALIZATION, AND EROTIZATION

Although there appears to be agreement that various affects can be experienced and "utilized" in a gratifying way, there is much confusion related to terminology. The three terms mentioned have been used interchangeably and in several frames of reference, an additional confusion.

Sexualization generally refers to the involvement of cognitive mental material, primarily fantasies with unconscious sexual meanings. For instance, sexualization of thinking in obsessive-compulsive neurosis permits a certain degree of self-gratification, but at the same time, because it brings this ordinarily conflict-free activity into the conflictual sphere, it may result in inhibition of it (Fenichel, 1945, p. 299). Hartmann (1955) equates sublimation with neutralization (desexualization and deaggressivation), and therefore considers sexualization a form of regression. He states that sexualized ego functions are subject to regressive tendencies. While sexualization usually refers to a function, or the nature of the transference, another use of the term relates to the use of an organ other than the naturally erotogenic ones for sexual gratification. Fenichel (1945) also spoke of "sexualization of non-sexual relationships," and discussed at length the possibility of inhibition of virtually every and any function which has become sexualized. He also refers to "sexualization of anxiety" (p. 483), but he limits this phrase to masochistic distortions in which fear or pain becomes a source of sexual excitement, a condition for genital sexual gratification.

The term "erotization" illustrates the problem, because it is sometimes used interchangeably with "sexualization" (as in "erotization of the transference"), and has been used in this sense by Freud (1926, p. 89), and sometimes as an equivalent to "libidinization" (LaForgue, 1930). And so, the fundamental question appears to be: "Is there a meaning to "libidinization" that connotes something different than sexualization?"

Fenichel, who used both terms extensively, seems to have thought so. In his essay on "The Defense Against Anxiety Particularly by Libidinization" (originally published in 1934), he deals actually not with a defense against *anxiety per se,* but against the *traumatogenic potentials* of it. But he is talking about "a defense against anxiety by developing libidinal pleasure in it" (p. 307). Note the use of the expression "libidinal pleasure." By using this expression, rather than just saying that people derive *pleasure,* he was glancing over and covering up a problem in this area.

The problem is that in the "libidinization" of anxiety or other affects, there is no sexual excitement, as there is for the perversions, nor is there necessarily a conscious quality of pleasure in it. This observation leaves us in a dilemma. We postulate a gratification in anxiety, and then we must add that this may happen without the conscious recognition of pleasure in the experience. This phenomenon *seems* to be perfectly well described and explained by the economic theory. In terms of the economic theory one would say that because of conflict, the conscious experience of pleasure is blocked, along with the repression of the "forbidden" fantasy or impulse, but this very defensive operation permits the anxiety (or other affect) to take over the discharge of instinctual energy, which was what was needed in the first place. This model has been used countless times since Freud described anxiety as a miniature hysteria (1926); it is what Fenichel referred to in calling it a "libidinal" pleasure rather than just pleasure. The more precise expression would be libidinal "gratification" since the conscious recognition of pleasure varies. It is precisely because this term lends itself to covering up the problem by "sweeping it under the carpet" of the economic-theory cliches that we must abandon its use. Instead of talking about libidinization, which always carries the risk of confounding us with thoughts of cathexes, let us simply consider shifts in the quality of pleasure related to an affect. We have many clinical observations to ponder. Observations abound about the extraordinary capacity for gratification which specific affects have for some individuals. Equally common are observations of people for whom the emotions that are usually pleasurable lose that quality and/or even become distressful.

How can we account for these common shifts in the gratification potential of affects without resorting to any allusion to the economic point of view of metapsychology? We know from clinical observations that the conscious awareness of pleasure in an affect may vary greatly, and may be virtually totally unconscious, even where this affect has become the only gratification available to the individual. How do we theoretically explain the psychic reality of those who bitterly complain of an affect experience or ego state which they are driven to produce in themselves with the compulsiveness of an addict? Our language simply has no provision for these developments. The defenses which necessitate the repression of conscious recognition of gratification in unpleasure and pain, the difficulties we have in admitting that certain assumptive gratifications are "not fun," also result in a general impoverishment of our language in this area. I will simply refer to the shifts in the quality of pleasure and/or distress attending the affective experiences. We must free our terminology regarding observational data from hypothetical valences. And in regard to these hedonic shifts, I am referring again to the *theoretically feasible situation in which there is a shift in its capacity for gratification, without the involvement of stimulation of an erotogenic zone.* There are some unanswered questions at this point. Does a shift in the capacity for gratification involve a change in the *quality of pleasure*? Can gratification and/or pleasure take place unconsciously? Since the consideration of these questions may involve a revision of the entire concept of what an affect is, let us consider some clinical observations in this area.

CLINICAL ASPECTS OF THE RELATION OF AFFECT TO THE QUALITY OF PLEASURE

When we think of the well-known examples which anxiety is experienced as pleasurable, as in an amusement park and in sports activities, we hasten to comment that the pleasure relates to the *mastery* of fear. When anxiety is associated with helplessness it may be experienced as distressful, but in association with other feelings – e.g., optimistic expectations, it is usually downright pleasurable. The following is an illustration of a "discovery" which became the precursor of what we usually call "libidinization of anxiety." Again, I must renounce this terminology and state only that, indeed, in this person there was evidence of considerable pleasure and gratification in experiencing anxiety in situations which did not involve helplessness.

A man of European background recalled in analysis that as a child (age six to twelve), living on the fifth floor of an apartment house, he had a curious pastime. He used to sit in the window facing the inner court in which there were usually a variety of activities. He found that he could lean out of the window to the point at which he would become frightened of falling out. He would either stay at this position or pull back just a bit, and then lean out again, producing within himself "bursts" of the feeling of anxiety. This activity did not have a compulsive nature, but it had a distinctly masturbatory quality, in the sense of a self-gratification devoid of any genital masturbatory stimulation. He simply learned to provoke his anxiety in a playful fashion; but only now, thirty years later, did he clearly realize that he did this for fun.

Upon considering the above clinical vignette, our thoughts drift practically automatically to the gratification involved in the *ideas* of falling which have such attraction. We are all very familiar with the kind of cognitive material which no doubt contributed to the fantasy gratification in this experience. But I must point out that the widely prevalent (among psychoanalysts) idea that thoughts, fantasies, or other cognitive acts are gratifying is mistaken. *An idea can be pleasurable only by mobilizing a reaction at an erotogenic zone, or a direct stimulation of hedonic centers of the brain, or by producing a pleasurable affect.* Thus, in the above case, if a fantasy was also involved, it resulted in some affective response. Also, if this individual had learned to think of, recall, or fantasize his "leaning-out-of-window experience" and was able to thus obtain the same response, it would not have been the *idea*, but the affective state which was perceptibly pleasurable. A major clinical fact hinges upon this consideration; that regardless of the fantasies involved, patients come to their doctors because they cannot tolerate the resultant affective states – and specifically the "expressive," physiological components of the affects and their distressful quality. When given medication the patients no longer mind their conflictual or previously anxiety-producing cognition.

Let us then return to my patient, who as a child made a remarkable discovery that he could produce anxiety within himself, and could keep it within bounds of comfort, and thereby devise a most remarkable and reliable means of self-gratification. It is a kind of "masturbation" which does not involve the stimulation of any of the usual erotogenic zones, for the locus of pleasure for him was somewhere deep in front of the lumbar and thoracic wall, where he experienced a tingling of the greatest pleasure he was capable of, similar to what he later experienced after an especially intense and gratifying orgasm, or at certain moments of dozing off. In respect to the capacity for gratification in an affect, every part of the body is an erotogenic zone. Thus, we have to distinguish pleasure in the *mastery* of an affect from the potential pleasure in *having* it.

Even in counterphobic behavior, with its compulsive nature, there is frequently a quality of pleasure (Fenichel, 1939). In contrast to the phobics, counterphobic individuals have a deep-seated conviction of their capacity to master the danger, and even the uncomfortable "expressive" aspects of affect. My impressions in this area are that when an individual discovers early a significant conscious pleasure in anxiety, he creates within himself a motivation and a tendency toward the counterphobic attitude which may carry the day, if at a future time he is confronted with a choice between attempting mastery or withdrawal and avoidance. The above-mentioned patient in later life showed a tendency to counterphobic and active mastery, as opposed to avoidance and passivity. However, even in those individuals who do develop phobic and avoidance patterns, in the advanced states of their analysis one finds a "core" of enjoyment and a high valuing of the anxiety. Anny Katan's report (1951) shows a clinging to the experience of anxiety in a case of an agoraphobic:

> It was amazing with what stubbornness my patient defended her agoraphobia . . . she clung to her anxiety desparately, and as the interconnections began to become clear to her, her anxiety concerned the loss of her anxiety. Whenever she was walking or standing, she had to make sure that she could still command her anxiety, she might stop because . . . this is what produced anxiety, then she would say to herself: "It'll come up, it'll come right away, immediately." If it did not turn up immediately or not intensively enough, she would predict the onset for the next street corner and would not give in until she again experienced the longed-for sensation. In her analysis, there occurred actual grotesque scenes; in moments of great excitement, she would wring her hands, and either scream or implore me with tears, "Please let me keep my anxiety, don't take it away." (p. 48).

The patient is pleading for the return of her precious anxiety, as a drug addict would for heroin. In fact, most addicts do crave the production of an emotion, mood, or consciousness modification at the same time they block another affect precursor (Krystal and Raskin, 1970). Hoppe (1962) has made the observation that survivors of Nazi persecution behave as if they developed a "hate addiction." Lifton (1963) has called a related phenomenon in the Hibakusha "survivor hubris."* But, as every psychoanalyst knows, ordinary childhood traumatization may produce similar disturbances which most commonly manifest themselves in our patients as gaining pleasure and gratification from anxiety which is also predominantly painful. Other affects can be libidinized in the same fashion.

Valenstein's (1973) study "On Attachment to Painful Feelings" contains a careful description of this process. His paper emphasizes the relation of attachment to pain as a function of early object relations – a most useful view which is confirmed in some of my cases, but which represents another aspect of the problem. It is remarkable that Valenstein, too, finds difficulty in the linguistics of gratification in painful affects. He speaks of "fixation to pain" (p. 373). He says: "for the most part this is psychic pain, although such patients do not emotionally neglect the possibility of *fulfilling themselves* with physically occasioned pain, should it present itself" (p. 365; italics mine). He refers to the painful "*Erlebniss*" as "paradoxically fulfilling even though not pleasurably or harmoniously satisfying" (p. 390). Perhaps poets and artists who have explored this painful bliss may help us out of the clinical linguistic paucity.

ART AND "TRISTIMANIA"

A phenomenon well worth a separate study is the appreciation of sadness, sorrow, and depressive suffering in the work and lives of many artists, poets, and writers, especially the romantic ones. Probably the most direct statement comes from Michelangelo who confessed (Sonnet #31, quoted in Wittkower, 1963, p.74):

*Melancholia is my pleasure and discomfort is my rest . . .**

---

* Hoppe et al. (1965) have also pointed out that problems of love or hate "addiction" are common in delinquent male adolescents. In the therapy of these youngsters, the addictive problems have to be approached as a specific issue.

Romanticist poets from William Blake and the *Sturm und Drang* of Schiller and early Goethe (*Die Leiden des Jungen Werthers*), through Chateaubriand, Lermontov, and Pushkin, and reaching the apogee in the lives and work of Shelley, Keats, and Byron, embraced and wallowed in their self-pity and misery as their most precious possession. Byron's Prisoner of Chillon declares: "I learn'd to love despair" (1816, p. 360). The rejoicing in sadness seemed to be the poetic predilection:

> *Go! You may call it madness, folly*
> *You shall not chase my gloom away!*
> *There is such charm in melancholy*
> *I would not if I could be gay.*
> (Samuel Rogers, 1914, p. 231)

Edel (1975) has borrowed a term coined by Benjamin Rush – "Tristimania" – to describe the thread of "madness in art," the themes of glorification of suffering, particularly the "mania of sadness" which he finds pervading "the works of great authors." As he puts it: ". . . nothing is more chronic among writers than their sadness" (p. 1007). He stresses, "Most artists would rather not be cured" (p. 19), and lists many examples of writers and poets who spent their lives in melancholy, which they treasured and poured into their art. He reports that Rilke refused psychoanalysis, saying: "Leave me my demons" (p. 1011).

But perhaps it should not really surprise us that a common characteristic of great art is that it beautifies, ennobles, elevates, and thus assuages the pain of those affects which are necessary for us to accept the realities of life. That artist is great who helps to mollify the painful affects attending everyday life, to become able to accept the existential tragedies of living. Hitherto, the discussion has viewed the affects as automatic and experienced passively. However, the observations of artistic expression remind us that, in fact, we are constantly involved in modifying and influencing our affective states. There is a kind of inhibition involved which causes us to disavow the fact of exercising control over affective and vital functions (Krystal,

---

* Dr. William G. Niederland, who had kindly brought this question to my attention, has pointed out that the word Michelangelo used for "pleasure" – "allergrezza" – is equivalent to "joy" or, in slang, "kicks," an implication very relevant to the further consideration of this paper.

1978a). Nonetheless, *the modification of the hedonic quality of affects may be considered one of the basic operations in affect tolerance.*

The effective manipulation of the hedonic aspect of emotions may be accomplished by "mixing" emotions or dealing with the aspect of helplessness or hopelessness in a situation of danger. Thus, to inspire hope or to deny the hopelessness of a situation will shift the anxiety toward the more optimistic and pleasurable side of the spectrum.

Affect modification need not always be motivated by pain avoidance and pleasure seeking. Like the poets, we sometimes choose to renounce excessive boisterousness or manic defenses against sadness and depression in order to attain a more profound, empathic, or wise view. Goethe stated this point explicitly:

> *Zart Gedicht, wie Regenbogen,*
> *wird nur auf dunklen Grund gezogen;*
> *darum behagt dem Dichtergenie*
> *das Element der Melancholie.*
>
> A tender poem, like a rainbow
> shows only against a darkened ground;
> therefore the element of melancholy
> suits the spirit of the poet.
> (Goethe, 1815, p. 73; translation mine)

Poetic expression becomes relevant when we turn our attention to the prevalence of these occurrences in everyday life. Benjamin Rush professed that poets "view the human mind in all its operations, whether natural or morbid, with a microscopic eye; and hence many things arrest their attention, which escape the notice of physicians" (quoted by Edel, 1975, p. 1006). At the same time, the poets and artists demonstrate that the pleasure of synthesis, functioning, performance, intellectual mastery, and playing may act as an effective balance to the distressful aspect of the "emergency affects," thus making them bearable (G. Klein, 1976). The playing of children lends the same kind of comfort, and is also endowed with beauty, order, harmony, and poise (Huizinga, 1950).

Thus, once alerted to changes in the quality of pleasure in affectivity, one discovers it to be quite a common occurrence. In many patients the manifestations of pleasure or gratification in painful feelings, or the anhedonia affecting their experience of pleasurable affects, are side issues, often overlooked. There are patients who have had "successfully" completed analyses who discover only later in life, when they are no longer able to distract themselves with their work, that their capacity for joy and pleasure and their capacity to feel the pleasure quality in affects as such is absent or severely diminished. Frequently, a serious depression develops at this point in reaction to their inability to experience gratification, in contrast to those patients who develop their anhedonia as a symptom of depression.

Conversely, some individuals freely use their imagination and their capacity to "look for the silver lining" when life is depressing. These are individuals with a good hedonic capacity. This function has been identified as a character trait by Meehl and colleagues (1971) who, using a term coined by Cattell (1935), have called it "surgency." These observations are easier to accept than the opposite – where the patients become attached to the maximization of a painful affect.

CASE ILLUSTRATION

Although virtually any affect may become the focus of modification of hedonic regulations, in some cases there may be a major shift in the pleasure and gratification role of a particular affect, most commonly, anxiety. Thus Valenstein (1973) speaks of patients "deeply attached to pain." In my recent experience I have had two patients who shared an attachment and gratification in anger, and two (surprisingly) who did the same with envy. Although the problems and difficulties involved were varied, these four patients had one thing in common: that at one point in analysis we discovered that the particular affect (anger and envy, respectively) was their secret way of getting their "kicks" out of life while other ways were blocked by inhibitions. The two patients with the "envy addiction" presented themselves with disparate problems – one with a tendency to depression and the other with overt homosexuality to which he continued to respond with distress. However, when the latter's behavior was observed, we found that what he was actually interested in was not homosexual gratification but approaching men, being refused, and then spending a lot of time nagging and feeling deprived.

The following is a vignette from the analysis of one of those patients who has enjoyed and treasured his anger:

On the occasion of his son obtaining a driver's license he went into a tirade against his own father who never taught him to drive, so that he had to do it on his own, at a later age, while other boys taught by their father got their license at 16. After the patient raged on for well over a half of the hour about how terrible his father had been, I brought his attention to his repeated need for this kind of outburst, which was especially inappropriate since he knew that his father had been schizophrenic, and since the father had now been dead for a number of years. This was part of his distortion designed to maintain the image of his father as *bad* (unwilling to teach his son) in order to continue his own rage. The patient became very angry with me, as if I had taken his father's place in a battle against him, and went on giving argument after argument as to why his father should have taught him to drive. Suddenly, he observed that he was defending his anger, and, in questioning himself about it, he discovered that his anger was precious to him and that he did not wish to give it up. He maintained a number of relations in his present life which he used to "feed" his anger, and was subject to fits of rage, many of them when alone, in which he yelled, screamed, raged on, and bit his fingers. His sessions regularly consisted in yelling at the top of his voice, until he reached a certain point of relaxation, after which he acted and felt sleepy.

This patient's uses of rage took up much work, as he frequently warded off other feelings, e.g., guilt or shame, by substituting anger. An identification with his anger, as indicated above, was also involved. Feeling *stronger* when angry thus also warded off feelings of dependence and helplessness. There was, in addition, in his case, a coupling of the rage with a feeling of deprivation which he used to justify an entitlement which, in turn, was the foundation of his life-style. After these and other uses and secondary gains in his rages were worked through, we ended up with the "purely gratificatory" use of anger. The pattern involved a number of things and issues over which he would get enraged constantly, for instance, lights being left on. On one occasion he came into his appointment with me and picked up a paper clip from the carpet. He then went on a harangue about people at his office constantly dropping used staples on the floor, and how he raged and screamed about it. When confronted with the fact that his experience of nineteen years of running the office has shown that staples will be found on the floor occasionally, he refused to accept it. Instead, he retained the expectation that whenever he saw a staple he *should* rage on – still justifying to himself that he was doing it in order to get people to stop dropping staples – even though this method had not worked in all these years. The outcome of this and a multitude of similar situations was that he was in a state of rage much of the time. The failure to accept the realities of the situation had a multitude of determinants, but his need to use anger for gratification was one of them.

Related to the hedonic aspects of affects are the vicissitudes of two sensations on the borderline of pleasure and pain: itching and tickling. In a presidential address to the American Medical Association section on Dermatology, Ayres (1964) discussed the "fine art of scratching" and reported that: "Scratching of normal skin will be felt as painful but scratching of equal intensity in an area of itchy skin produces erotic pleasure, hence the presence of a particular excitatory state has the effect of transforming an ordinarily painful stimulus, scratching, into a source of erotic pleasure" (p. 1005).

I am indebted to Dr. William Niederland for a vignette of a case involving tickling. His patient was tickled as a child by his older brother. The experience started each time as a very pleasant and exciting one but would regularly go on to such length and intensity that it became unbearably painful, and the patient feared that the brother would kill him by continuing the now terrifying stimulation. Niederland commented that the German word *Totlachen* referred to the general fear of mirth reaching similarly unbearably intensity, with sadomasochistic excitement getting out of control.

The above observations on itching and tickling illustrate just how radically the quality of pleasure and distress may shift in a given experience. The same is true with affects in situations where the affect remains the same, but the quality of pleasure is shifted. This action may be mediated by blending of affects or other affect modification, e.g., mirth turning to sadness. The very idea of humor turning pain into pleasure is a related operation. But for our purposes it is important to emphasize the "pure" modifications or shifts in the hedonic quality of affects. These changes need not be permanent. Once alerted to the possibility of shifts in the quality of pleasure in affectivity, one discovered that there is considerable variation within a given individual. Each affective experience, each feeling, is a blend of elements, among which the hedonic quality is an independent variable. Since we are not used to such an idea in psychoanalysis, we may borrow a model derived from neurophysiology and neuroanatomy which suggests a separate derivation of the pain and pleasure experience and its intimate association with the general emotional apparatus.

THE PLEASURE AND DISTRESS CENTERS: THE USE OF ANATOMY AS A METAPHOR OF PSYCHIC FUNCTION

Hitherto the models used for the conceptualization of psychic pleasure have been in the idea of discharge modeled after the male ejaculation, mistaken with the idea of orgasm, and the idea of foreplay.* The demonstration by Olds, Milner, Delgado, Miller, and others that there are pleasure and distress centers of the brain opened a new view of pleasure (Olds and Miller, 1954; Delgado, Roberts and Miller, 1954; Olds and Olds, 1963). The centers for pleasure and distress are closely associated with the limbic system related to emotions (MacLean, 1949), but are separate and distinct from it. The pleasure centers have their own extensive "pathways of reward" which extend to the frontal cortex, the hypothalamus, the pontine tegmentum, and the medula. The medial forebrain bundle is a "pleasure relay station" for the other brain pathways (Routtenberg, 1978, p. 160). There is also an area in the cerebellum, connected with both the pleasure and distress centers, which functions in such a way that stimulation of it blocks the distress and pain areas and, simultaneously, stimulates the pleasure centers. Heath (1977b) has demonstrated that a variety of otherwise untreatable disorders can be treated by implanting a brain pacer in this cerebellar site. The importance of such a single action, which simultaneously assuages bad feelings and promotes good ones, is that it provides the model for which we are searching. Certainly we must find a way to explain the shifts in the hedonic quality of affects in a *single operation*. The new physiological and pharmacological studies now give us the answer in the form of hormones which have an endogenous opiatelike effect. The endorphins and enkephalins *simultaneously* relieve pain while granting a sensation of pleasure as well as counteracting the "arousing" effect of emotions and pain, and hence fulfill our requirements (Goldstein, 1976; Guillemin, 1977)."†

Heath's studies on the pleasure and distress centers and their relation to emotional function and mental illness have been inspired by the views of his teacher, Sandor Rado, who was convinced that "the pleasure economy" was essential in regulating behavior and object relations (Heath, 1974). Rado (1964, 1969) felt that the hedonic regulations were the major factor in emotional and mental illness. The discovery of the group of brain hormones concerned with hedonic regulation is an exciting confirmation of these views.

---

* In this regard there has always been some fuzzy thinking, since the ejaculation per se has been confused with the emotional "discharge."

† There is also a peptide which is not blocked by opiate antagonists: Neurotensin. Snyder (1980) has reviewed the mind-boggling multiplicity of polypeptide neurotransmitters, which link the hedonic regulation with a multitude of visceral, affective, and vital functions and provide for a complex interaction between the affective and hedonic states and the homeostatic functions of the organism.

While anatomically and neurophysiologically there are two distinct centers – one registering pleasurable sensations and the other distress – in terms of the psychic reality of an adult, the experience is more of a spectrum which endows each mental event with a quality of relative pleasure or distress. Although the genetic history of this development is as yet little known, an *attenuation* of the intensity of the pleasure (and distress) experience seems to take place, so that the psychological effect in the adult is to make the impact less intense.

The demonstration of the existence of pleasure and distress centers, as well as a whole system of neurotransmitters involved in the regulation of pleasure and distress, necessitates that we provide a psychological framework for their function. We must create theories and proceed with studies of the psychological consequences of the development and function of these biological regulations of the hedonic aspect of mental function; particularly the hedonic aspect of affects, and their consequences to the nature and function of the mind. But the use of anatomy and physiology in this work is strictly *metaphoric*. Anatomy and physiology illustrate my clinical impression that there may be a derivation of the hedonic quality of affects separate from the other aspects and attributes of emotions. Raskin and I earlier discussed the clinical implications of the view that the experience of pain was not a simple perception, but a complex experience (Krystal and Raskin, 1970). The demonstration of the pleasure and distress centers being discrete from and connected to the limbic system suggests that, similarly, the affect experience should be considered to be a composite.

In addition to the cognitive aspect of an affect (the meaning of it), there is the "expressive" part. This part of affect is subjectively closely associated with the experience of pleasure or distress, as if the latter were an inherent part of the emotion. However, both the anatomical and clinical observations suggest that the quality of pleasure of affect is quite separately derived, and only associatively linked with a particular affect.* The association and the result produced are the same as when one perceives his mother's face and experiences joy. The joy is not identical with the perception. Nor is the pleasure or distress in the emotion identical with the emotion.

---

* In addition to the hedonic one, a fourth element of affects is suggested by physiological studies: it is likely that the activating or tonically mobilizing quality of emotions also has a separate source and variability (Mandell, 1970).

The observations on changes in the experience of pleasure of anxiety and other affects and the addictive uses of some affects by my patients suggest that the shifting of the hedonic quality of affects is fairly common. This shift can be achieved voluntarily as well, through imagining an appropriate scene and other techniques (Krystal, 1978a). We may now return to some of the questions posed previously. It seems that gratification may take place unconsciously, because pleasure, like guilt or other affective experiences, may occur but not be consciously registered. The possibility of either pleasure or pain occurring without conscious registration is best demonstrated by an experiment in hypnotic analgesia in which the subject denied experiencing any pain while his automatic writing was filled with exclamatives and requests to stop the torture (Hilgard, 1974).

These unconscious gratifications or distresses are clinically noticeable in their actions as motivators – as in the problem of an unconscious sense of guilt or what I referred to above as "affect addictions." What we have reviewed also suggests that the perception and conscious registration of the hedonic quality of affects may be shifted, suppressed, or magnified defensively. It may also be modified by association with other affects, as illustrated in the poetic "ennobling" of existential despair. Most of all, the very intensity of the pleasure or distress experience can be modified, as seen by these clinical illustrations of changes in the hedonic quality of affects. It is necessary to distinguish the variation in conscious *registration* of gratification (or distress) from the variation in the gratification (or distress) experience itself.

In fact, we can now accept as a basic premise, based on the work of research hypnotists, primarily Hilgard (1974; Knox, 1974) that we must separate the conception of pleasure from gratification, and suffering from pain, as these are capable of separate variations. Moreover, we must acknowledge that all four qualities, as well as a multitude of combinatorial experiences (such as the combined pleasure, pain, gratification and distress in itching) may register in various degrees of consciousness and various degrees of self-sight.*

Moreover, as D. Klein points out in this volume (See Chapter 1), we have to distinguish appetitive motivation and activities from

---

* The expression "self-sight" has been coined by Lawrence P. Tourkow, M.D. in 1953 to denote that only those experiences which are consciously recognized to be a part of one's self-representation are free from repression and therefore apt to be utilizable in one's self interest.

consummatory ones. This view doubles the number of combinations of hedonic regulatory possibilities. We now have to account for (and we can utilize for the understanding of our clinical observations) the possibility of pleasure or gratification, pain (distress) or suffering in regard to both appetitive and consummatory principles, and in the broad scope of conscious registration. For it is clear that the question of the quality of conscious registration of affect, and especially its hedonic quality, cannot be accurately approached by the "conscious or unconscious" duality – but rather seen in a spectrum of experiences.

While I have emphasized the hedonic shifts in affects, probably the most common experience is that the patient's hedonic capacity is low – or secondarily lowered (Meehl, 1975). Of course, these conditions are quite familiar to us in the form of various anhedonic states, particularly depression. However, not even in depression can we safely assume that there is an anhedonia proportional to the severity of depression. Fawcett and associates have demonstrated (1983) by clinical studies, in following up a hunch by D. Klein (1974), that only <u>some</u> depressed patients are significantly anhedonic. Still, at least some depressive affective states can significantly alter the hedonic regulation. There are also situations when sexual excitement becomes distressful, or when any other proleptic (gratification-expecting) affect is experienced as uncomfortable or painful. Studies in severe posttraumatic states suggest that the most common after-effect lies in the diminution in the capacity for pleasure and joy, a state of anhedonia which may represent a permanent alteration of these functions (Krystal, 1978b).

IMPLICATIONS OF HEDONIC SHIFTS FOR PSYCHOANALYTIC TECHNIQUE

In regard to the counterphobic attitude, Fenichel (1945) observed: "the counterphobic individual can engage pleasurably in the activity which he originally feared, if during the procedure he demonstrates to an object with whom he is unconsciously identified that he is protecting or pardoning it" (p. 169). In this example Fenichel is talking about a kind of manipulation, which secondarily produces a shift in the pleasure modality of an affect. By finding protection symbolically, the individual diminishes the perception of helplessness in a situation of (subjectively perceived) danger. But the "true" counterphobic continues to have anxiety while carrying out the dreaded act; only he learns to enjoy the anxiety.

How does this happen? A few things could be considered. If the counterphobic activity leads to later pride and self-confidence, a "foreplay" element could be in effect. As Jacobson (1953) put it: "The expectation of future gratification appears to induce pleasurable components which we are entitled to call signal affect too, though of a pleasurable variety" (p. 64). While that view may explain the "pleasurization" of anxiety in certain sexual activities, as in "forbidden games," it could hardly be the whole answer in counterphobics, because for them the mastery never takes place, and the individual merely denies this potential insight.

It will be helpful to return to the consideration of masochism at this point. In the masochistic perversion, pain becomes *sexualized.* It becomes part of the necessary conditions which permit genital sexual gratification, and so it assumes a role similar to a fetish, in the sense that it affects the subjects in a way parallel to perceiving sexual characteristics. Just as an average man might find any aspect of a woman's body "exciting," because it signals potential sexual gratification, so in the perversion, the pain or the actual or symbolic manifestations of sadism in the potential partner takes the place of the usual erotic stimulus. But the dependence upon the stimulation of the genitals and producing a sexual gratification remains.

Not so in moral masochism. If moral masochism exists at all, then we assume that usually painful affects such as shame, despair, or others now become pleasurable or a source of gratification. There is, of course, also a hidden "gain" for the masochist who by making himself a victim avoids the self-confrontation with his guilt over sadism; but this is a negative quality. The moral masochist avoids greater pain, but the question is from where does he derive his gratification? The motivation in this shift was originally defensive in nature, and in our analytic work we have to identify these defenses, and the underlying infantile unconscious fantasies. When the patient can work with these, he may find that he can dispense with the defenses. But in addition, we must take into account the "natural history" of this kind of disturbance; namely, that the patient has learned to take pleasure in a previously painful affect, related to a masochistically exhibitionistic activity of displaying himself in a castrated condition. *This development has to be dealt with directly* by interpreting the shifts and pointing out their consequences.

Once the therapist conceives of the possibility that gratification may not be derived from pleasure, but rather from pain, and that *all* the hedonic experiences may register unconsciously or in a repressed form, a whole world opens up for further exploration and intervention.

Thus it may be found that some obsessive-compulsives desire gratification from their self-attacks and depressive mood production (wallowing in sadness). When one elucidates these mechanisms one finds a virtual addiction to such forms of self-gratification.

The clinical relevance of the above observation lies in the fact that if an ordinarily painful affect becomes gratifying, the patient gains a secret and frequently *not consciously recognized* source of gratification. No matter how accurate all the other interpretations are, he is not about to give up this secret, most valued possession. Thus the "pleasurization" of an affect constitutes a motivation for resistance which prevents any changes in his emotional makeup and function. This resistance has to be interpreted, and the patient's gratification in and valuing of his "bad" feelings have to be confronted as a major analytic task. The interpretation and working through of affect goes beyond the work with neuroses, for it often addresses itself to preverbal development. Only in working through these attachments can the associations of affects with the experience of pleasure be shifted. In this respect our work consists of a double task. On the one hand, the patient has to give up pleasure in an affect or activity hitherto enjoyed. On the other hand, he has to dare to try to explore the affect or activity which he has heretofore experienced as prohibited to him, and gradually learn that *he may do it* (or have it) and then that he may *enjoy it*. He then may be able to establish associative links of it with enjoyment and, as a final step, consciously admit to himself that he enjoys it. Thus, as analysts we pay attention to the psychic reality of a patient who is given a chance to discover for himself the defensive values of his past behavior and accomplish an active mastery of his change, having resolved the related conflicts.

CASE ILLUSTRATION

One of the previously mentioned patients had shown homosexuality with an underlying problem of libidinization of envy, as well as a narcissistic personality disturbance and several other types of difficulties. As he progressed in his analysis, he discovered that his lack of interest in women was defensive in nature and secondary to his giving up of his masculine ambitions because of castration anxiety. While till now he kept protesting that he had nothing to offer a woman (because he had only one testicle), he finally dared to approach a woman other than a prostitute and had a successful sexual experience. Consequently we discovered that his homosexual activities were designed to provide a kind of gratification which was a "secret" from himself. His "kicks" were derived out of evoking intense envy in himself, and demonstrating that the "perfect" individuals rejected him and considered him worthless. There would be produced a "bouquet" of dysphoric affects involving helplessness, shame, and self-pity but also a white-washing of his guilt (since he was a victim, and therefore innocent, rather than hateful, revengeful , greedy, etc). To this consciously painful, but vaguely recognizable, gratifying experience he was addicted.

Once this secret gratification was exposed and explored in terms of its historical, epigenetic derivations, and the multitude of fantasies involved, we found that an enormous creativity was involved in that the development of these behavior patterns made his survival possible. Upon the thorough exploration of the defenses, conflicts and impulses involved, there finally came the question of whether he'd be prepared to give up his secret self-gratification. Here we came to the part of the problem which makes me refer to these problems as "addictions." The point was that, as in substance dependence, the drug use represents an attempt at problem solving and self-soothing or self-stimulation and, although it miscarries, the patient is still loathe to give up the only thing that he has found dependably helpful. So this patient demonstrated that most extraordinary stubbornness and defiance by maintaining that the patterns developed were "him," and that he was resigned to live his life as a miserable wretch retaining his secret gratification.

There were, in this case, two separate processes mentioned before: (1) the perversion in which sexual excitement was shifted from genital activity with the use of genitals, to the use of the mouth, with masturbation as a *secret* source of gratification, "officially" disavowed. (2) The experiencing of gratification in the emotions of envy, shame, attachment to painful feelings, and the negative therapeutic reaction.

I was, in fact, the third therapist in this case; an analyst and a psychiatrist had worked with this patient for many years. However, it was not possible to deal with the perversion without first enabling the patient to restore the usual associations of joy with his accomplishments and with his successes, and renouncing, very gradually, his gratification in affects usually considered distressing.

Once we can separate in our minds the pleasure attribute of an affect, we can observe shifts in the usual pattern, and then can turn to the use of the usual psychoanalytic technique to discover their genetic background. They will be found to be defensive, and will sometimes yield to psychoanalytic therapy. This is the clinical advantage of the conception of affect as a composite.

PLEASURE AND DISTRESS SIGNALS IN THE INFANT

Lastly, we return to the question of hedonic functions in the infant which provide the signals necessary in the formation of self- and object representations. As I stated previously, our genetic studies on affect tell us that the young do not have signal affects available to them because these are attained only by maturation. Yet, as far as we can determine, the early object and self-perceptions are dominated by their pleasurable or distressful quality. We must therefore postulate two types of hedonic signals. The "adult type" is indeed derived from the maturation of our affects, and becomes available in our "affective memory circuits" as signals. Through the complex association the affective aspect of every mental event provides a qualitative dimension to it. Part of this affective experience is a "flavor," as it were, of *pleasure or distress* or a mixture of these. As adults, we experience ourselves most of the time in the midline of this scale, and at such times we do not register the conscious awareness of an emotion. Most of our operations are carried out with such minimal quantities of affect responses that we are hardly aware of them. However, the hedonic quality, which has through the epigenesis become intimately associated with every affect, determines the subjective nature of every self and object representation.

In the infant, however, in the absence of signal affects, the direct experience of pleasure and distress, the "naked," as it were, activation of the pleasure and aversive centers provides that signal function. This is one of the reasons why in early life the hedonic quality of the perception of the object carries such an enormous weight. Thus we are dealing with a pure *pleasure and distress signal*, something that is not observable in the adult, because of the intimate association of this response with the other aspects of affects.

June Hadley (1984) has demonstrated that indeed, such functions could be envisioned by the consideration of the theories of the amygdala as an amplification-registration system, working in an integrated fashion with the hippocampal error-eliminating system.

Moreover, Hadley demonstrated that the human infant was "preprogrammed," as it were, to register and become sensitized to the mother's voice in the third trimester of pregnancy, and that the above-mentioned anatomical units could be understood to provide a pleasurable experience when the infant recognizes the mother's voice, when he or she registers the perception of a face – particularly if that face becomes familiar, expected, and is offered for the child to use in his own natural rhythms of attention and inattention. Thus Hadley's work (1984) seems to confirm my anticipation that a hedonic evaluation of early object perception must be available before affects have developed to a point where they are available as signals.

Stern (1983) has surveyed a number of direct infant observations which further demonstrate that a gratification (reward) system is operating since birth, and that learning theory is applicable as an explanation of preferences for the mothering parent as registered through various senses.

The early registrations of pleasure and distress are coded through the phylogenetic makeup of the newborn. The responses relate mostly to the vital functions of the infant; nutrition and elimination, and (in mammals), a need for an intimate physical relationship with the mother. It is this primitive self-reward and self-punishment system that takes the place of the signal affect in the infant. It functions in the same way as signal affects, as we understand them in adults, but it is devoid of the complex background of memories and modifications. George Klein (1976) worked out the functions of the "vital pleasures" without resorting to the use of the economic point of view. He stressed that the enjoyment of the sexual experience of infancy was probably "an important primary source of affiliation and attachment" (p. 222). He also re-emphasized Harlow's (1958) contribution relating the "contact comfort" to the pleasures of sensual arousal.

The associative modifications *mollify* the intensity of the pleasure and distress experiences, which by comparison to adults are quite intense, if not violent, in the infant. The implications of this postulate will, of course, require further exploration and consideration.

SUMMARY

Our subjective experience seems to indicate that affects can be classified in two major categories: pleasurable ones like joy and distressful ones like fear or anger. We therefore tend to assume that the quality of pleasure is an inherent part of an emotion. However, psychoanalysts have long known that under some circumstances, emotions such as anxiety may take over the function of gratifications, when the normal channels are blocked by intrapsychic conflict. In an attempt to explain such phenomena in terms of the economic theory, such conditions are called "libidinization" of an affect, e.g., anxiety, with the indication that the affect derived its pleasurable nature by virtue of facilitating drive-energy discharge. The concretization of these metaphors has led to the erroneous idea that the cure for affective disturbances was the "excretion" of these affects, as if they were noxious substances.

In the present study, the neuro-anatomical findings that there are pleasure and distress centers distinct from, but closely associated with, the "emotional brain" are considered in parallel to our clinical observations. This view indicates that the quality of pleasure or distress is not an inherent part of the affect experience, but one associatively linked. In certain clinical conditions, the quality of pleasure usually associated with a given affect may be shifted, and emotions usually experienced as pleasant may become painful, while in others, usually unpleasant affects may become the major mode of obtaining "kicks" in life. In posttraumatic situations, there is a suppression of the capacity to experience pleasure and joy; the resulting anhedonia is a reliable "marker" of such states.

These findings further indicate that in the exploration of emotions we need to identify the several elements such as the cognitive and expressive ones. We also have to look out for the vicissitudes of the associated responses which provide dimensions which are normally intimately connected with given emotions, namely, the hedonic quality and the tonic activating property. Only when all of these exist simultaneously, and the subject recognizes this fact, through reflective self-awareness, does he have a "feeling." Feelings are the optimal adult signal affect, characterized by their availability in low intensity when they are most easily recognized as signals to one's self. In the infant, in the absence of signal affects, the direct action of the pleasure and distress center provides a powerful and predominant signal. As the hedonic function becomes associatively linked with the other aspects of affect, the impact of the pleasure and distress signal upon the self is softened. This makes it more useful and more manageable.

REFERENCES

Ainsworth, M.D. (Salter), Blehar, M.D., Walters, E. and Wall, S. (1978). *Patterns of Attachment*. Hillsdale, N.J.: Lawrence Erlbaum.

Bowlby, J. (1969). Attachment and loss. In J. Bowlby (Ed.), *Attachment*, Vol I. New York: Basic Books.

Fawcett, J., Clark, D.C., Scheftner, W.A. and Hedeker, D. (1983). Differences between anhedonic and normally hedonic depressive states. *Arch. Gen. Psychiatry*, 40:1027–1030.

Freud, S. (1926). Inhibitions, symptoms, and anxiety. In J. Strachey (Ed. 1959), *The Standard Edition of the Complete Psychological Works of Sigmund Freud.* London: Hogarth Press.

Goethe, J.W. (1815). Sprichwortlich. In *Gott, Gemueht und Welt*, vol. 2 of *Complete Works*. Munich: Deutscher Taschen buch Verlag.

Goldstein, A. (1976). Opioid peptides (endorphins) in pituitary and brain. *Science*, 193:1081–1086.

Greenspan, S.I. (1981). *Psychopathology and Adaptation in Infancy and Early Childhood.* New York: International Universities Press.

Guillemin, R. (1977). Endorphins, brain peptides that act like opiates. *New Eng. J. Med.*, 296:226–228.

Hadley, J., (1984). *Attention, Affect and Attachment.* Manuscript in preparation.

Harlow, H. F. (1958). The nature of love. *Amer. J. Psychol.*, 13:673–685.

Hartmann, H. (1955). Notes on a theory of sublimation. *The Psychoanalytic Study of the Child*, 10:9–29.

Heath, R. G. (1974). Application of Sandor Rado's adaptational psychodynamics formulations to brain physiology. *J. Amer. Acad. Psychoanal.*, 2:19–25.

Health, R.G. (1977). Modulation of emotion with a brain pacemaker. *J. Nerv. Ment. Dis.*, 165:300–317.

Hilgard, E. R. (1974). Divided consciousness in hypnosis: The implications of the hidden observer. In E. Fromm and R.E. Shor (Eds.), *Hypnosis: Developments in Research and New Perspectives*, 2nd ed. New York: Aldine.

Hoppe, K. (1962). Persecution, depression and aggression. *Bull. Menninger Clin.*, 26:195–203.

Hoppe, K., Molnar, J., and Newell, J. E. (1965). Love and hate addiction in delinquent male adolescents. *Psychother. Psychosom.*, 13:271–277.

Huizinga, J. (1950). *Homo Ludens: A Study of the Play Element in Culture.* Boston: Beacon Press.

Jacobson, E. (1953). The affects and their pleasure-unpleasure qualities in relation to psychic discharge processes. In R.M. Lowenstein (Ed.), *Drives, Affect, Behavior.* New York: International Universities Press.

Katan, A. (1951). The role of "displacement" in agoraphobia. *Internat. J. Psycho-Anal.*, 32:41–50.

Kernberg, O. F. (1976). *Object Relations Theory and Clinical Psychoanalysis.* New York: Jason Aronson.

Kernberg, O.F. (1982). Self, ego, affects and drives. *J. Amer. Psychoan. Assoc.*, 30:893–918.

Klein, D. (1974). Endogenomorphic depression: A conceptual and terminological revision. *Arch. Gen. Psychiat.*, 31:447–454.

Klein, G.S. (1976). The vital pleasures. In G.S. Klein (Ed.), *Psychoanalytic Theory.* New York: International Universities Press.

Knox, J. V., Morgan, A. H. and Hilgard, E. R. (1974). Pain and suffering in ischemia. *Arch. Gen. Psychiat.*, 30:840–847.

Krystal, H. (1974). The genetic development of affects regression. *Annual of Psycho analysis*, 2:98–126.

Krystal, H. (1975). Affect tolerance. *Annual of Psychoanalysis*, 3:179–219.

Krystal, H. (1978a). Self-representation and the capacity for self-care. *The Annual of Psychoanalysis*, 6:209–246.

Krystal, H. (1978b). Aspects of affect theory. *Bull. Menninger Clin.*, 41:1–26.

Krystal, H. and Raskin, H. (1970). *Drug Dependence.* Detroit: Wayne State University Press.

Krystal, J. H. (1984). Animal Models of Stress and Depression: Mechanism of Illness and Recovery. Unpublished manuscrpt.

Laforgue, R. (1930). On eroticization of anxiety. *Internat. J. Psycho-Anal.*, 11:312–321.

Lifton, R. J. (1963). Psychological effects of the atomic bomb in Hiroshima - The theme of death. *Daedalus*, 92:462–497.

MacLean, P. D. (1949). Psychosomatic disease and the "visceral brain." *Psychosom. Med.*, 11:338–358.

Mandell, A. J. (1970). Neurochemical considerations relevant to human affective states. In J. Masserman (Ed.), *Depression: Theories and Therapies.* New York: Grune & Stratton.

Meehl, P. E., Lykken, D.T., Schofield, W. and Tellegen, A. (1971). Recaptured item technique (RIT): A method for reducing somewhat the subjective element in factor naming. *J. Exper. Research on Personality*, 5:171–190.

Meehl, P.E. (1975). Hedonic capacity: Some conjectures. *Bull. Menninger Clin.*, 30:295–307.

Olds, J. (1958). Self-stimulation of the brain. *Science*, 127:315–324.

Olds, J. and Milner, P. (1954). Positive reinforcement produced by electric stimulation of septal area and other regions of rat brain. *J. Compar. Phys. & Psychol.*, 47:419–427.

Olds, J. and and Olds, M. E. (1963). Approach avoidance analysis of rat diencephalon. *J. Comp. Neur.*, 120:259–295.

Parkes, M. D. and Stevenson-Hinde, J. (1982). *The Place of Attachment in Human Behavior.* New York: Basic Books.

Pribram, K. H. (1968). The new neurology and the biology of emotions: A structural approach. *Amer. Psychologist,* 22:830–838.

Rado, S. (1964). Hedonic self-regulation of the organism. In R. Heath (Ed.), *The Role of Pleasure in Behavior.* New York: Harper & Row.

Rado, S. (1969). Adaptational psychodynamics: Motivation and control. In *Emotions.* New York: Science House.

Rogers, S. (1914). In D. Sargent (Ed. 1960), *The Complete Poetical Works of Samuel Rogers.* Boston: Crosby, Nichols, Lee & Co.

Routtenberg, A. (1978). The reward system of the brain. *Scientific American,* 239:154–165.

Snyder, S. H. (1980). Brain peptides as neurotransmitters. *Science,* 209:976–983.

Stern, D. (1983). Implications of infancy research for psychoanalytic theory and practice. In L. Grinspoon (Ed.), *Psychiatry Update Vol. II.* Washington: American Psychiatric Press.

Valenstein, A. F. (1973). On attachment to painful feelings. *The Psychoanalytic Study of the Child,* 21:365–392.

Wittkower, R. M. (1963). *Born under Saturn.* London: Weidenfield & Nicholson.

Wundt, W. (1920). *Grundriss der Psychologie,* 2nd ed. Stuttgart: Engelmann.

8

Anhedonia and Alexithymia: A Potential Correlation?

PETER E. SIFNEOS

One of the questions raised by the topic of this volume has to do with the differentiation between anhedonia and alexithymia (Sifneos, 1972). Before proceeding to deal with this complex question, I should like to describe alexithymia briefly since all readers may not be as familiar with this concept as they are with anhedonia.

Alexithymia was conceptualized in the mid-1960s after systematic clinical observation of some patients suffering from a variety of classic psychosomatic diseases (Sifneos, 1967). It can be defined as a deficiency in the ability to connect emotions with fantasies. This deficiency in a patient's ability to cope with emotions has similarities to the memory defect which one encounters in patients suffering from Korsakoff's syndrome.

The main characteristics of alexithymia involve an impoverished fantasy life and marked difficulty using appropriate words to describe emotions (Sifneos, Apfel-Savitz et al., 1966). This is precisely what the word alexithymia means (from the Greek a"lack, lexis"work, thymos"emotion). Also, there is a tendency to describe endless and trivial details surrounding an event which was likely to arouse emotions (this has been labeled by the French analysts as "pensee operatoire") (Marty and de M'Uzan, 1963). In addition, there is an urgency to act, a tendency to assume rigid postures and a diminished capacity to cry and to dream. Confusion also seems to prevail in the patient's ability to distinguish between different emotions, as well as to feel emotional in thinking about a past event which might have given rise to emotions. Finally, alexithymic individuals seem to be unable to point to various parts of the body where emotions are being felt.

During a clinical interview with an alexithymic individual, the evaluator is struck by the patient's inability to initiate conversation, and by his preference to answer questions laconically, yet at the same time the patient gives the impression that he frantically wants to communicate but is unable to do so due to his alexithymic defects. An analogy may be made between the alexithymic patient and the color-blind individual who is asked to describe a color which he is unable to see. The resulting frustration is reflected in the patient's inability to communicate, and the observer is struck by the efforts which are being made by the patient to parrot words depicting emotions used by the interviewer without really being able to understand clearly the meaning of these very words.

In addition to these major deficiencies, alexithymic patients tend to have physical complaints which they describe in detail and which on many occasions are totally unrelated to the underlying pathology of any disease from which they might be suffering. In sum, these alexithymic characteristics point to a basic inability on the part of the patient, as mentioned already, to connect their emotions with their fantasies.

At this point it may be helpful to turn our attention and attempt to understand the biopsychosocial aspect of emotions. Ever since Cannon's (1915, 1932) establishment of the physiology of emotion as a central thalamic homeostatic mechanism which at times of emergency utilizes autonomic and endocrine circuits for the expression of fight or flight, there has been a major effort to understand the biological side of emotions by a variety of other investigators. Starting with Kluver and Bucy (1939), experimental work on primates and carnivorous animals and observations on humans have led us to believe that structures in the limbic system, like the amygdaloid complex and the hippocampus through their command of the hypothalamus, and the pituitary, and their connections with the autonomic nervous and endocrine systems, play a key integrating role in visceral emotional balance (Duty, 1967; Bear, 1983).

MacLean's description (1948) of a "triune brain" (reptilian, limbic, and neomammalian) offers an interesting way to view alexithymia (MacLean, 1977; Hoppe, 1975). All three are involved with emotions but it is not clear exactly how they intercommunicate. One possibility has to do with the biochemical coding devices. It is certainly clear, however, that they do not use words to integrate among each other. It is possible therefore that if one may assume that defects may exist in the communication of reverberating circuits between the limbic and the neommamalian brain, alexithymia is likely to be the result.

If such a breakdown in communication were to take place, then the reptilian and limbic brain systems with their automatic and endocrine expressions (i.e. "visceral emotions") will have no neocortical-thalamic representation which is responsible for a conscious awareness recognized by humans as a "feeling."

The Greek work for feeling ("synaesthema") clearly points to a dual component: "biological" (aesthema) "plus" (syn) neocortical cognitive activity accompanying it. Thus it may be assumed that "affect" has both a biological and a cognitive component to it, and the resulting emotions can be either "visceral" or "feeling" ones. A feeling then may be defined as a visceral emotion which in addition has a cognitive component in terms of the fantasies which accompany it.

In discussing the neuroanatomy and neurophysiology of emotions, one should also emphasize the role played by the two cerebral hemispheres. For example, it has been reported that patients who had commissurotomies also developed alexithymic characteristics (Hoppe, 1975). Although it is a well-known fact that the left hemisphere is associated with speech in right-handed individuals, recently it has been shown that the right hemisphere is not only dominant for many emotional functions but also plays a major role in coloring, giving special intonation, and generally modulating the affective component of speech. Furthermore, it is of interest that lesions in the right brain produce pathological laughter, while lesions in the left brain give rise to uncontrollable crying (Ross and Mesulam, 1979; Ross, 1981; Ross and Rush, 1981).

If we return now to the discussion of the neocortical activity attached to visceral emotion which gives rise to feelings, it should be emphasized that appraisal and knowledge of previous experience are important processes which help us recognize and evaluate incoming sensations (Arnold, 1960). These in turn are registered and compared by means of memory with similar situations in the past labeled as "good" or "bad." It is possible that they may give rise to appropriate action. It should also be added that the social setting in which all this activity takes place may also determine whether a given state may be viewed as being "pleasant" or "unpleasant."

Labeling, however, is strictly influenced by two key factors: the understanding of the meaning of the previous experience, and the language that is used to express it. Difficulties in both of these areas can appear if lesions are present in the right hemisphere as has already been mentioned. For example, if incoming sensations reach the limbic system and give rise to visceral emotions but cannot arouse appropriate neocortical activity in the form of fantasies due to genetic or biological defects, then two possibilities are likely. The first one would give rise to cortical activity inappropriate to the visceral emotion; that is, a description of endless details relating to environmental stimuli but not fantasies connected to the visceral emotion. This is what the French psychoanalysts call "pensée opératoire," when, for example, a patient who has been insulted describes all the details surrounding the situation in which he found himself and the action which he took, but is unable to use the word "anger" to describe his emotion and denies having any fantasies associated with it. The second possibility has to do with an absence of any neocortical activity but instead a resulting autonomic and/or endocrine hyperactivity.

Clinically, alexithymia, as mentioned already, was first observed in some individuals suffering from a variety of psychosomatic diseases. However, this is not the case in all psychosomatic patients. It has also been shown that individuals who are alexithymnic may not necessarily be ill or that they may possess characteristics of alcoholic, drug-addicted or sociopathic individuals. The possible explanation for all these clinical findings may lie in the presence or the absence of defects existing in the peripheral organs and determining the symptom formation of the underlying psychosomatic diseases. For example, defects present in the stomach of an alexithymic patient with absence of fantasies and autonomic hyperactivity could lead to the development of peptic ulcer, while defects in the synovial membranes, bronchioles, colon or arterioles could account for the development of symptoms of rheumatoid arthritis, asthma, ulcerative colitis, or hypertension.

As far as those drug addicts or alcoholic patients who are also alexithymic, one may visualize such individuals as having felt progressively more tense as a result of their deficiencies in the area of feelings. Furthermore, living in a feelings-saturated society, and being unable to recognize, appraise and process them verbally, they may utilize a short cut to relieve this tension and may drink alcohol or take excessive amounts of drugs and thus become addicted to them. In the same way an alexithymic sociopath who has observed the effect that certain feeling words have for other people, yet is unable to understand the real meaning of these words, may use words such as "love," "joy," and "happiness" with great effectiveness in his interpersonal relations without being able to experience them or without their having the slightest impact on his own behavior patterns.

At this point it should also be added that two types of alexithymia have been described: "primary" and "secondary." In the former, the alexithymic characteristics are thought to be due to structural or neurobiological defects. Secondary alexithymia, on the other hand, is viewed as resulting from developmental arrests, or from a catastrophic environmental onslaught upon the patient. Finally, one may also consider the classic psychoanalytic explanation that these defects are due to an excessive use of denial and repression. Analytically, these secondary alexithymic patients are thought to be able to verbalize and to fantasize, but not to have learned to pay attention to their feelings or are not willing to utilize these capabilities which they nevertheless possess.

ANHEDONIA

If we now turn our attention to anhedonia, we are again faced with the need to define the term "hedone" or "pleasure." This is not an easy task. Hedone, in addition to its biopsychosocial component, has a philosophical dimension to it which has preoccupied mankind for more than two millenia. Since the days of the Greek philosopher Epicouros (Epicurus, Latin) and his school, much controversy has revolved around the ethics of "hedone." In Epicurian terms, sensation was the sole criterion for "good" or "bad," and hedone was viewed as the be-all and end-all of life. In addition a distinction had been made between "active hedone" (such as joy) and "passive hedone" involving an absence of pain ("aponia") or lack of anxiety ("ataxia"). This Epicurian view of hedone is clearly an individualistic philosophy in contrast to the perspective of Hume, who added to the word "pleasure" a social component. Keeping in mind the distinction between "active" and "passive" hedone, one should also be reminded that pleasure has a neuroanatomical site in the midbrain, limbic system, and hypothalamus of lower animals. In humans, however, there is in addition a neocortical component, both psychological and social.

In psychoanalytic terms, Freud viewed pleasure as a lowering of tension and as a diminution of excitation, which he referred to as the "ego" or the "death" instinct, and which in the final analysis leads to total extinction. In contrast, he conceptualized a "sexual" instinct which he viewed as leading to procreation and renewal of life.

One may then equate the "active hedone" of Epicouros with the "sexual instinct," of Freud, in contrast to the "passive hedone" or the "death instinct," which involves absence of pain and diminution of tension (Freud, 1920). In addition this "active hedone" or "pleasure" can be viewed as a true "feeling" as it has already been defined with a neuroanatomical site and an additional neocortical component to it in the form of pleasure-giving fantasies. This neocortical aspect helps us to recognize and evaluate pleasurable sensations, appraise them appropriately by comparing them with previous pleasant experiences, use language to label them, and action to express them.

Fantasies can give rise to pleasant feelings by helping one visualize, anticipate, and experience pleasure. Furthermore, a rich fantasy life helps us to entertain ourselves and not to become dependent on others for entertainment for receiving pleasure. In addition, fantasies serve a role in alleviating painful experiences. An individual, therefore, who is unable to utilize pleasant fantasies efficiently because of an absence of fantasies, a high threshold potential to fantasize, or an inability to use appropriate fantasies and language to deal with a painful event, and who is therefore unable to extricate himself from a painful experience, will complain endlessly and talks at length about the details surrounding it (pensée opératoire) without being able to describe the impact that it may have upon him.

Since anhedonia has been defined as an "insensibility relating to pleasure alone," and since pleasure has been defined as true "feeling," then an anhedonic individual who (due to genetic variables which give rise to his low hedonic threshold or other reasons) is unable to connect his fantasies with the visceral pleasure-giving emotions should also be viewed as alexithymic (Fawcett, Clark et al., 1983). If anhedonia, however, is due to a depressive mood, then the anhedonia may also disappear once the depressive episode remits. Therefore, an anhedonic individual may or may not be alexithymic, while an alexithymic individual is always anhedonic.

In the case of the alexythimic anhedonic patient who has been treated by antidepressant medication and is not depressed anymore, the anhedonia should persist despite successful therapy. The antidepressant medication will affect only the biology of the depressive mood, but it cannot provide the patient with the pleasant fantasies (which are either absent or are not connected with the visceral pleasurable emotions).

One may conclude that anhedonia, primary alexithymia, and endogenous depression are of biological origin and require anti-depressant medication for the relief of the depression. One should not expect, however, that there would be any change in either the anhedonia or the alexithymia. Furthermore no dynamic psychotherapeutic intervention would be expected to help these individuals because this therapy tends to increase tension, and patients who are treated in this way remain unchanged or become worse off. This has been the case with patients suffering from chronic ulcerative colitis studied by Karush, who were described as being "obtuse, passive and having symbiotic tendencies." These patients were obviously alexithymic and the majority did poorly after they received psychoanalytic psychotherapy (Karush et al., 1969). It also seems clear that only supportive or anxiety-suppressing kinds of psychotherapy should be offered to depressed anhedonic and primary alexithymic individuals.

If, on the other hand, anhedonia, secondary alexithymia and depression co-exist, then the psychotherapeutic interventions dealing with the secondary alexithymic characteristics will necessitate the use of a specialized kind of dynamic psychotherapeutic technique. Such a therapy has been advocated by Krystal, who attempts to teach the patient how to pay attention to his own fantasies, how to learn to improve his affect tolerance and how to use appropriate words to verbalize them (Krystal, 1979). Another approach with the alexithymic depressed anhedonic patients may be Wolf's attempt to teach them how "to play" since they seem to have "lost their ability to play" and enjoy life. Such patients may also be treated with antidepressant medication.

One of the difficulties which we have at the present time has to do with a valid measure of alexithymia. Although the Beth Israel Questionnaire has been thought to be a useful measuring tool, it still may be subject to inter-rater bias since it is the interviewer who scores the patient (Sifneos, 1973). Patient self-report questionnaires such as the Schalling Sifneos, the SAT 9, and the modified MMPI are also fairly reliable, but unfortunately none is clearly the perfect instrument. Thus it is important to continue efforts to develop a reliable measure of alexithymia because early diagnosis will facilitate appropriate antidepressant treatment and proper psychotherapeutic care (Apfel and Sifneos, 1979).

Anhedonia and alexithymia are difficult subjects to contemplate and to study. Nevertheless, by correlating neurobiological, psychological, and social factors these concepts do offer exciting possibilities for research in some of the most perplexing aspects of human behavior (Cobb, 1950).

REFERENCES

Apfel, R. and Sifneos, P.E. (1979). Alexithymia concept and measurement. *Psychotherapy and Psychosomatics*, 32:180-191.

Arnold, M.B. (1960). *Emotions and Personality*, Vol. II. New York: Columbia Univ. Press.

Bear, D.M. (1983). Hemispheric specialization and neurology of emotion. *Archives of Neurology*, 40:195-203.

Cannon, W. (1915). *Bodily Changes in Pain, Hunger, Fear, Rage* (2nd ed.). New York: Appleton.

Cannon, W. (1932). *The Wisdom of the Body*. New York: Norton.

Cobb, S. (1950). *Emotions and Clinical Medicine*. New York: W.W. Norton Co. Inc.

Doty, W. (1967). The nerve, impulse and synaptic transmission. In A.M. Freedman and H.I. Kaplan, *Comprehensive Textbook of Psychiatry*. Baltimore: Williams & Wilkins.

Fawcett, J., Clark, D.C., Scheftner, W.A., and Gibbons, R.D. (1983). Assessing anhedonia in psychiatric patients. *Arch. Gen. Psychiatry*, 40:79-85.

Freud, S. (1920). Beyond the pleasure principle. In J. Strachey (Ed. 1959), *The Standard Edition of the Complete Psychological Works of Sigmund Freud*. London: Hogarth Press.

Hoppe, K.D. (1975). Liaison psychiatry and psychoanalysis. In R.D. Pasnau (Ed.), *Consultation-Liaison Psychiatry*. New York: Grune & Stratton.

Karush, A., Daniels, G.E., O'Connor, J.F. and Stein, L.O. (1969). The response to psychotherapy in chronic ulcerative colitis. *Psychosom. Med.*, 31:201-227.

Kluver, H. and Bucy, P.D. (1939). Preliminary analysis of functions of the temporal lobes in monkeys. *Archives of Neurology and Psychiatry*, 42:979-1000.

Krystal, H. (1979). Alexithymia and psychotherapy. *Amer. J. Psychotherapy*, 33:17-28.

MacLean, P.D. (1949). Psychosomatic disease and the "visceral brain." *Psychosomatic Medicine*, 11:338-353.

MacLean, P.D. (1977). The triune brain in conflict. *Psychotherapy and Psychosomatics*, 28:207-220.

Marty, P. and de M'Uzan, D.C. (1963). *L'Investigation Psychosomatique*. Paris: Presses Universitaires.

Meehl, P.E. (1975). Hedonic capacity. *Bull. Menninger Clinic*, 39:295-308.

Ross, E.D. (1981). The Aprosodias. *Arch. Neurol.*, 38:561-570.

Ross, E.D. and Mesulam, M.M. (1979). Dominant language functions of the right hemisphere. *Arch. Neurol.*, 36:144-149.

Ross, E.D. and Rush, P.A. (1981). Diagnosis and neuroanatomical correlates of depression in brain-damaged patients. *Arch Gen. Psychiatry*, 38:1344-1355.

Sifneos, P.E. (1967). Clinical observations on some patients suffering from a variety of psychosomatic diseases. *Acta Med. Psychosom.*, 7:1-10.

Sifneos, P.E. (1972). *Short-Term Psychotherapy and Emotional Crisis*. Cambridge, Mass.: Harvard University Press.

Sifneos, P.E. (1973). The prevalence of alexithymic characteristics in psychosomatic patients. *Psychotherapy and Psychosomatics*, 22:255-263.

Sifneos, P.E., Apfel-Savitz, R., and Frankel, F.H. (1977). The phenomenon of alexithymia. *Psychotherapy and Psychosomatics*, 28:47-57.

9

Cellular Basis of Positive Reinforcement

LARRY STEIN
JAMES D. BELUZZI

The phenomenon of positive reinforcement is well established at the level of the whole animal. If a response is closely and regularly followed by a reinforcing stimulus, the behavior is strengthened or its probability is increased. A behavioral response obviously reflects the activity of many neurons. Is it the integrated activity of these neurons that is reinforced; that is, is reinforcement exerted at the level of neuronal systems? Or is it the individual activities of the relevant neurons that is reinforced; that is, is reinforcement exerted at the cellular level (Klopf, 1982)?

It is commonly believed that reinforcement is exerted at the systems level. According to this view, the reinforcement of behavioral responses is paralleled at the neuronal level by the strengthening or reorganization of complex neuronal circuits or assemblies (Hebb, 1949). Unfortunately, no such circuit or cell assembly for any reinforced behavior has yet been identified. Where in the rat's brain, for example, would one find the circuit for a lever-press response? And how would one measure the changes in circuitry that are induced when lever-pressing is reinforced? These anatomical and physiological considerations, as well as difficulties at the behavioral level associated with response definition, have led some psychologists to ask whether it really is correct to say that the whole response is the functional unit for reinforcement. According to Skinner (1953), a more useful conceptual scheme assumes that all responses are made up of elements, and that it is these elements or "behavioral atoms" (p. 94), and not whole responses, that are the units strengthened by reinforcement. If so, and if atoms of behavior can be represented by the activity of individual neurons, then positive reinforcement may actually occur at the level of individual cells, as suggested by Klopf (1982).

The cellular hypothesis suggests an analogy between reinforced behavior and an ant colony. If you watch an ant colony from a distance as it descends on a pile of sugar, it looks much like one large creature moving towards the sugar. However, close up, the colony is seen to be no single creature, but rather an aggregated mass of individual ants. In the terms of the analogy, the important question for a theory of reinforcement is, who tastes the sugar? Obviously it is not the ant colony as a whole, but the individual ants themselves that actually taste the sugar. Similarly, it could be argued that in the brain it is the behavior of individual neurons, and not the integrated activity of neuronal circuits, that is directly modified by reinforcing signals.

Olds (1965) was the first to report apparent evidence for the operant conditioning of single neurons. In these experiments, rats with implanted microelectrodes received food or rewarding brain stimulation contingent on appropriate bursts of single-unit activity. Firing rates were increased in a number of cases, suggesting reinforcement of the single-unit response. Unfortunately, it is not clear whether it was the behavior of the individual neuron that was being reinforced or whether some more complex response or movement, of which the neuron's activity was a part, actually was being reinforced. In some of Olds' tests a restriction system was used to limit movement: electronic detectors were discharged by most movements and these precluded reinforcement. Although operant conditioning was still obtained under these conditions, one cannot rule out the possible reinforcement of behaviors involving undetected movements, such as postural adjustments or attentional responses. Like other investigators who have attempted to demonstrate operant conditioning of single-unit activity (Fetz, 1969; Wyler and Robbins, 1980), Olds recognized that, if a reinforcing stimulus is delivered to a behaving animal, it is impossible to separate the reinforcement of single units from the reinforcement of more complex responses.

One solution to this problem is to deliver a reinforcing stimulus only to the neuron being conditioned. But what is effective reinforcement for a single neuron? According to the catecholamine-endorphin theory (Stein, 1978; Stein & Belluzzi, 1979), reinforcement signals normally are delivered to their neuronal targets by the release of catecholamines or endorphins. If so, it might be possible to duplicate these natural signals of reinforcement by the direct application of the transmitters to appropriate neurons. In such experiments catecholamines or endorphins would be applied via micropipettes to individual units in various regions of the brain following particular rates or patterns of activity. These rates or patterns should be strengthened only by contingent application of the transmitters, and not by noncontingent application.

METHODS

Surgery and Brain Slice Preparation

In whole brain experiments, rats were anesthetized with chloral hydrate, artificially respirated, and placed in a stereotaxic instrument. A micropipette was lowered into different brain regions through a small hole in the skull, and slowly advanced until suitable action potentials were displayed on the oscilloscope. In brain slice experiments, rats were decapitated, and their brains were rapidly removed (30-45 sec) and chilled to 6° C in oxygenated artificial cerebrospinal fluid (ACSF; Dingledine et al., 1980). Using plastic tools, the hippocampal region was dissected out and rinsed repeatedly with cold ACSF to minimize cell damage. A 4-mm block was isolated by parasagittal cuts using a tissue chopper. One cut end of the block was glued with cyanoacrylate to the bottom of the cutting chamber and supported by surrounding it with agarose (1.8%, 43° C). Once secured, the tissue was again immersed in ACSF at 6° C and further sectioned with a vibratome to yield about six 400-μ slices. The slices were individually transferred to a static chamber and supported on nylon mesh at the surface of ACSF solution in an oxygenated atmosphere (95/5 O_2/CO_2, 500 ml/min) at 35° C. At least 1 hour of incubation was allowed for recovery of physiological activity prior to the start of experiments (Schwartzkroin, 1981; Teyler, 1980). Fresh ACSF was infused into the static chamber every 30-45 min.

Extracellular Recording and Pressure Microinjection

Single-barrel micropipette blanks (Omega Dot) were pulled and back-filled with test solution or vehicle (165 mM saline). The micropipette was connected to a pressure injector, and the tip broken back under microscopic control to produce a droplet 18 μ in diameter at an injector setting of 15 p.s.i. and 35 ms. Using a micropositioner, the micropipette was visually guided to targeted cells and slowly lowered until a suitable action potential was obtained. Unit activity was displayed on a digital storage oscilloscope, monitored on a loud speaker, and recorded on a strip chart recorder. Important criteria for the selection of suitable cells included a signal/noise ratio of at least

4:1 and relatively stable levels of baseline activity. Action potentials were led into an amplitude analyzer, whose output provided digitized input to the computer and to a rate/interval analyzer. Firing rates were displayed on a strip chart recorder. Minicomputers were programmed to count unit activity, activate the injection pump, store data on- line and analyze data off-line. A 7-channel FM recorder provided a permanent record of all essential experimental events in sequence for later analysis.

A high-pressure microinjection system was used for rapid extracellular delivery of picoliter volumes of neurotransmitters and drugs. Pressure injection is required for immediate delivery of reinforcing solutions with injection durations as short as 5 ms. High pressure nylaflow tubing was used to connect the injection pump to the micropipette.

Single-Unit Operant Conditioning Procedures

A somewhat arbitrary decision was made in choosing which aspect of unit activity to reinforce. Since firing rates are likely to be an important vehicle for information transmission, peak rates should have high information value and might be amenable to conditioning. Thus, in these experiments, we defined a half-second period of relatively fast activity as the neuronal response to reinforce. These neuronal responses or "bursts" were individually determined for each unit studied. Prior to the start of conditioning, 500 successive half-second samples of neuronal activity were recorded and a frequency distribution of the number of spikes per sample was compiled. A "burst" was defined as that spike number that was equalled or exceeded in only 2 percent of the samples.

The basic operant conditioning method involved six states: 1) *Baseline*. The number of "bursts" in the absence of reinforcement (operant level) was determined during a baseline period of approximately 10 minutes. 2) *Operant Conditioning*. Each "burst" was now followed by an injection of the reinforcing solution. If conditioning failed to occur after 5 minutes, the duration of the injection (and hence the dose) was increased until evidence of conditioning was obtained, or until direct pharmacological or mechanical effects interfered with recording. 3) *Extinction*. Reinforcement was terminated, and recording continued until the baseline was recovered. 4) *Matched "Free" Injections*. Noncontingent injections of the reinforcing solution were made at regular intervals to determine direct pharmacological effects on rates of firing and probability of "bursts." The pattern and number of "free" injections were matched to the pattern and number of reinforcing injections in the preceding phase of operant conditioning. The presentation of programmed free injections was delayed for three sec after the occurence of "bursts" to minimize their adventitious reinforcement. 5) *Washout.* A second baseline period without injections was given to allow residual effects of the noncontingent drug administrations to be dissipated. 6) *Reacquisition.* Whenever possible, a second period of reinforcement was scheduled in order to compare rates of original acquisition and reacquisition.

RESULTS

Whole Brain

Initial work was performed in the whole animal to maximize the probability of successful experiments. In the absence of experience with locally applied reinforcement, it was felt that surgical reduction of the preparation, or the use of cells in culture, should be deferred until positive results could be demonstrated in the intact brain. An early positive experiment in an intact, anesthetized preparation with cocaine (a dopamine enhancer) as the reinforcing solution is displayed in Figure 9.1. This unit, probably located in dorsal hypothalamus, exhibited a seven-fold increase in the number of "bursts" and a two-fold increase in overall firing rate following approximately 20 cocaine reinforcements. The same number of free cocaine injections had no effect on the number of "bursts" or overall spike frequency. Another apparently positive experiment with amphetamine (a dopamine releaser) as the reinforcing agent is shown for a unit presumably located in hippocampus (Fig. 9.2). In this case, a dramatic increase in the rate of "bursts" observed after approximately 6 reinforcements. Twenty similar amphetamine injections, administered noncontingently in the free injection phase, produced no significant increase in the number of "bursts" or overall spike rate. Introduction of an FR-2 schedule caused a decline in "bursts" in this and other experiments. Reintroduction of the regular reinforcement schedule increased the number of "bursts" which again decreased when the FR-2 schedule was reinstated. A similar experiment with the dopamine receptor agonist apomorphine serving as the reinforcing drug is shown for a unit presumably located in the reticular nucleus of the thalamus (Fig. 9.3). In this case, an increase in injection duration from 70 to 100 ms was required for evidence of operant conditioning. Free injections of apomorphine, both preceding and following the reinforcement phase, failed to increase the number of "bursts" or the overall spike rate above baseline, suggesting that direct stimulation cannot explain

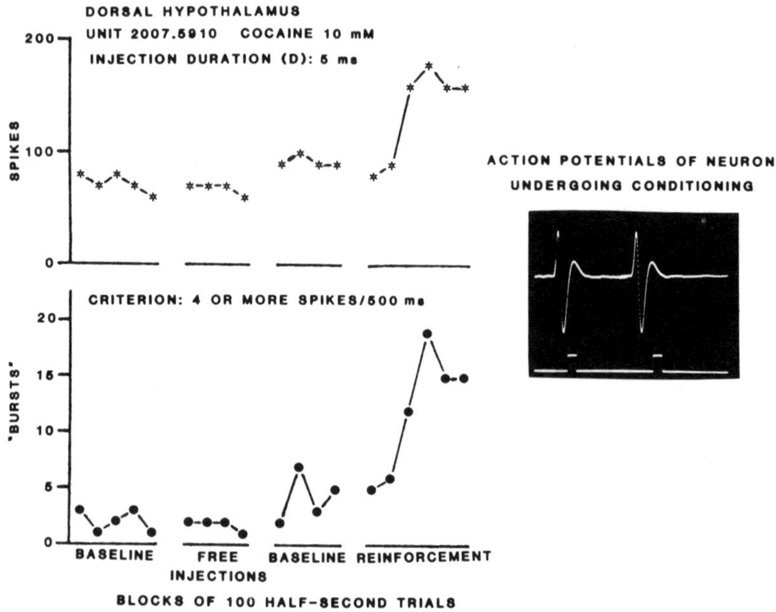

Figure 9.1. Operant conditioning of a neuron in rat brain presumed to be located in dorsal hypothalamus using local injections of cocaine as reinforcement. Unit activity throughout four phases of a complete experiment is shown. Prior to the first baseline phase, the "burst" criterion of 4 or more spikes per half-second sample was established. Each point shows the number of "bursts" (lower graph) and number of spikes (upper graph) in blocks of 100 half-second samples or trials. In the second phase, free injections of cocaine HC1 (10 mM in 165 mM saline) were made after every 20th half-second trial for a total of 20 free injections. The injection duration was 5 ms. Following a second baseline period, the 5-ms duration cocaine injections were delivered after each "burst" (reinforcement phase). "Bursts" and overall spike rate were increased by the contingent cocaine injections during the reinforcement phase, but were not increased when the same injections were administered noncontingently in the free injection phase. Inset: (upper trace) photograph of digital oscilloscope display of two action potentials from the unit undergoing conditioning, and (lower trace) 1-ms time markers.

apomorphine's reinforcing action. Finally, a negative control experiment, in which saline was substituted for the reinforcing drugs, is shown in Figure 9.4. No evidence of operant conditioning was observed, suggesting that a chemically specific message, and not the mere contingency of pressure microinjection following bursts, is required for reinforcement.

Brain Slices

Contrary to initial expectation, our most satisfactory experiments have been performed in brain slices. This reduced preparation isolates the cell undergoing conditioning from many of its normal

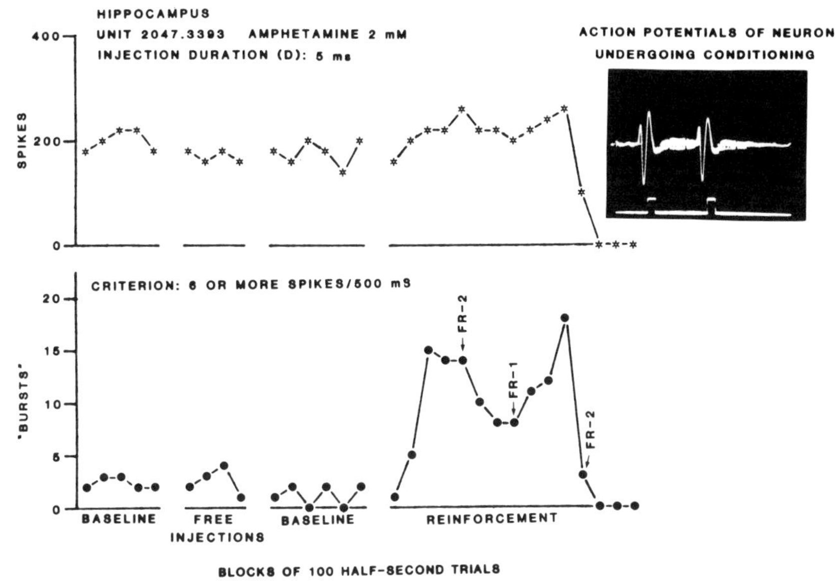

Figure 9.2. Operant conditioning of a presumed hippocampal neuron in rat brain using local injections of amphetamine as reinforcement. For details, see text and Fig. 9.1. FR-1 = regular reinforcement schedule, FR-2 = fixed-ratio 2 reinforcement schedule.

connections. Use of brain slices furthermore eliminates the artifacts associated with anesthesia and the possibility that, even under anesthesia, animals may be influenced by environmental stimulation. Still another major advantage of the brain slice technique is the ability to return to the same cell type from experiment to experiment since microelectrode placement is under direct visual control. At present we have focused our efforts on hippocampal slices, aiming our micropipettes at the large pyramidal cells in the CA1 field of dorsal hippocampus.

A positive experiment using dopamine as the reinforcing solution is shown for a hippocampal unit in Figure 9.5. The frequency of "bursts" and overall firing rates were rapidly increased after approximately 10 reinforcements in two separate phases of operant conditioning. The same dopamine injections administered noncontingently failed to increase either "burst" frequency or overall firing rate. It may also be noted that extinction occurred rapidly following both instances of operant conditioning. A second positive experiment using cocaine is shown in Figure 9.6. An initial period of free injections delivered at a rate of approximately 5 per minute had no effect on the

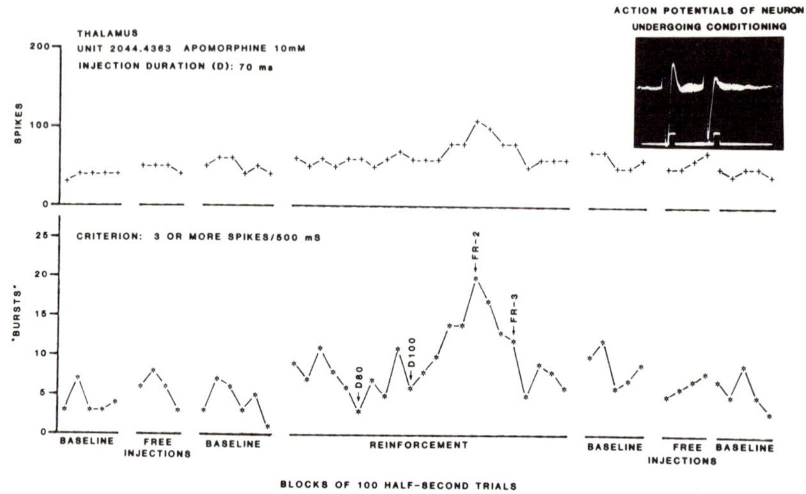

Figure 9.3. Operant conditioning of a presumed thalamic neuron in rat brain using local injections of apomorphine as reinforcement. For details, see text and Fig. 9.2. At D80 injection duration increased from 70 to 80 ms, at D100 injection duration increased from 80 to 100 ms. FR-2 = fixed-ratio 2 reinforcement schedule, FR-3 = fixed ratio 3 reinforcement schedule.

frequency of "bursts" or on overall firing rate. During a first phase of operant conditioning, "bursts" and firing rates were sharply increased after approximately 10 applications of cocaine. Extinction following the first phase of reinforcement initially produced a high rate in "bursts" and spike frequency, but then a sharp decline. Free cocaine injections again were given in a second phase, at the rate of approximately one every 5 seconds to match the peak rate obtained in the preceding reinforcement phase. These densely packed free injections had no effect on the number of "bursts" or the overall firing rate. In a second phase of operant conditioning, contingent injections of dopamine again increased the frequency of "bursts" and overall firing rate, but not to the level observed in the first phase of reinforcement. In control experiments, dopamine was administered noncontingently throughout the experiment (Fig. 9.7) or saline was substituted for dopamine (Fig. 9.8). In neither case was "burst" frequency or overall firing rate increased. We have also observed that effective doses of reinforcing solutions in hippocampal slice experiments seem to be

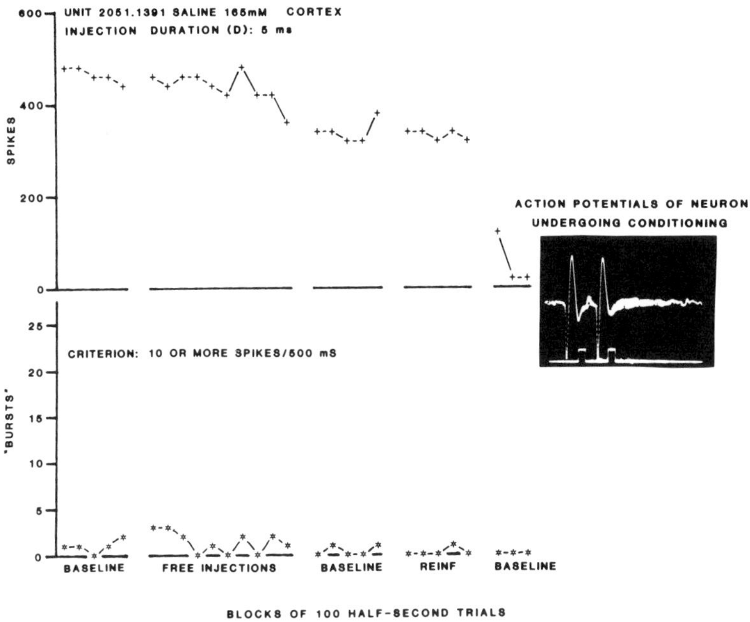

Figure 9.4. Saline control experiment. Failure to obtain evidence of operant conditioning of a presumed cortical neuron in rat brain using local injections of saline as reinforcement. For details, see text and Figure 9.2.

lower by an order of magnitude than those in whole brain experiments.

A summary of 8 positive experiments is shown in Figure 9.9. Plotted here are the means of the peak rates obtained in each phase of the experiment for each neuron. Highly significant increases were obtained in each of the reinforcement periods when compared either to control periods or periods when the dopamine was presented independently of neuronal bursting. A similar summary of the positive cocaine experiments is shown in Figure 9.10.

Finally, all hippocampal slice experiments containing useful data are summarized in Table 9.1. Excluded from this table are the many experiments in which suitable action potentials could not be obtained or held, or in which artifacts, such as drug overdoses or clogging of the micropipette, caused experiments to be abandoned. In the columns labelled "RESULTS", the designations are as follows: + = conditioning-like changes (increased probability of bursts following reinforcement) plus noncontingent controls, ? = conditioning-like

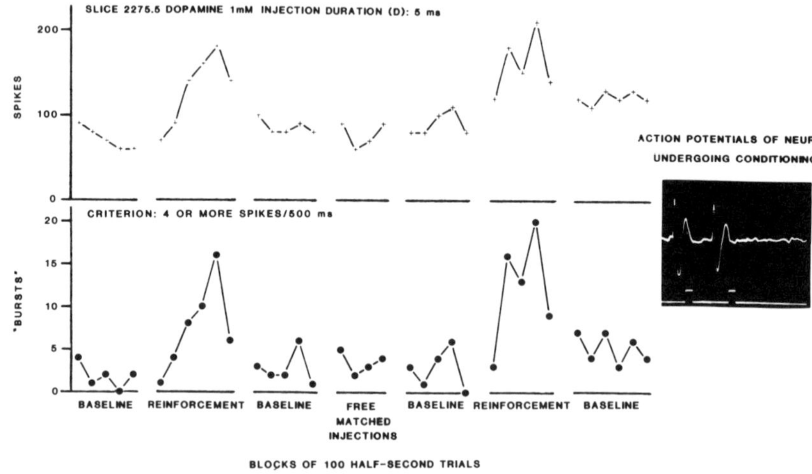

Figure 9.5. Operant conditioning of the activity of a CA1 pyramidal cell in a slice of dorsal hippocampus using local injections of dopamine as reinforcement. The activity of the unit throughout seven phases of a complete experiment is shown. Each point shows the number of "bursts" (lower graph) and the total number of spikes (upper graph) in successive blocks of 100 half-second samples or trials. Prior to the first baseline phase, a "burst" criterion of 4 or more spikes per half-second sample was selected; this criterion gave a "burst" rate for this unit that never exceeded 4% in the initial baseline period. In the reinforcement phase, dopamine HC1 (1 mM in 165 mM saline) was applied for 5 ms immediately after each "burst." Following a second baseline period, the same dopamine injections were delivered independently of the unit's behavior as a control for possible stimulant effects: the number of injections were matched to those "earned" during the last four periods of the reinforcement phase. "Burst" and overall spike rates were increased by the contingent dopamine injections during the reinforcement phase, but were not increased when the same injections were administered noncontingently in the free matched injection phase. Inset: (upper trace) photograph of digital oscilloscope display of two action potentials from the unit undergoing conditioning, and (lower trace) 1-ms time markers

changes but no controls, and – = no evidence of conditioning. The table thus indicates that 9 of 17 completed dopamine experiments were positive and contained noncontingent controls. In the cocaine experiments, the success rate was substantially lower than in the dopamine experiments. We do not know the explanation, but speculate that cocaine, which acts via dopamine, may require a physiologically active dopamine system to exert its full reinforcing effect. Since the dopamine axons are severed in the hippocampal slice preparation, it is conceivable that their responsivity to cocaine is reduced.

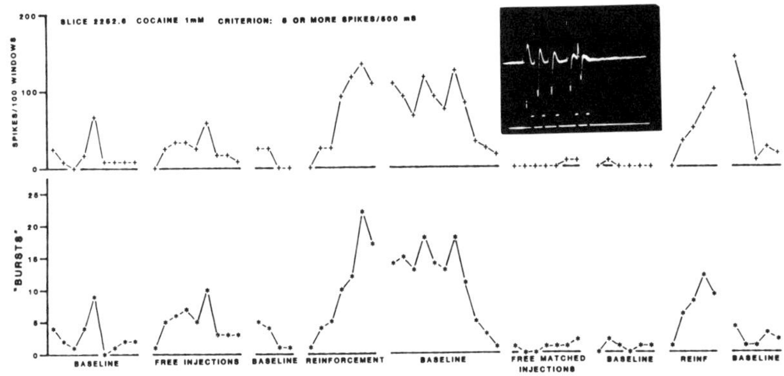

Figure 9.6. Operant conditioning of a pyramidal neuron in a dorsal hippocampal slice using local injections of cocaine as reinforcement. For details, see text and Figure 9.5.

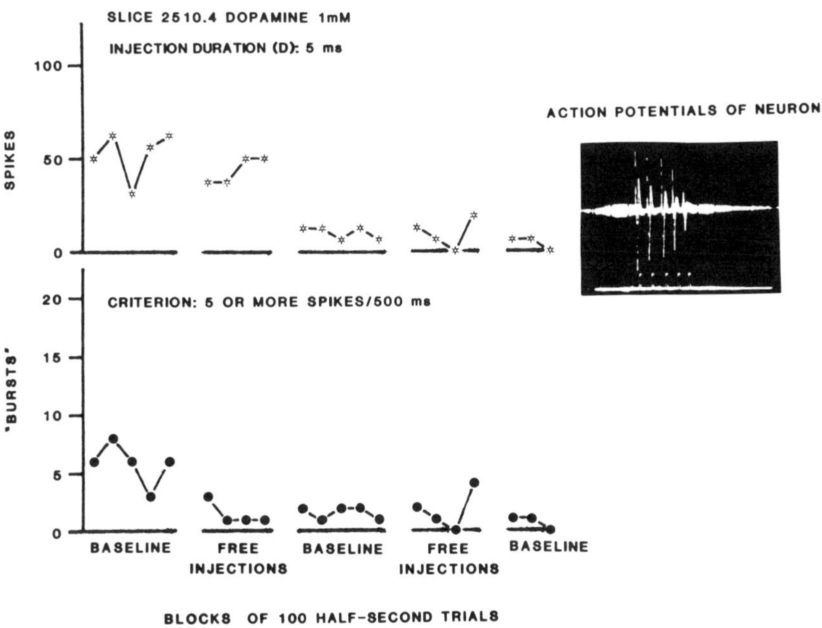

Figure 9.7. Control experiment with dopamine administered noncontingently to a pyramidal neuron in hippocampal slice. For details, see text and Figure 9.5

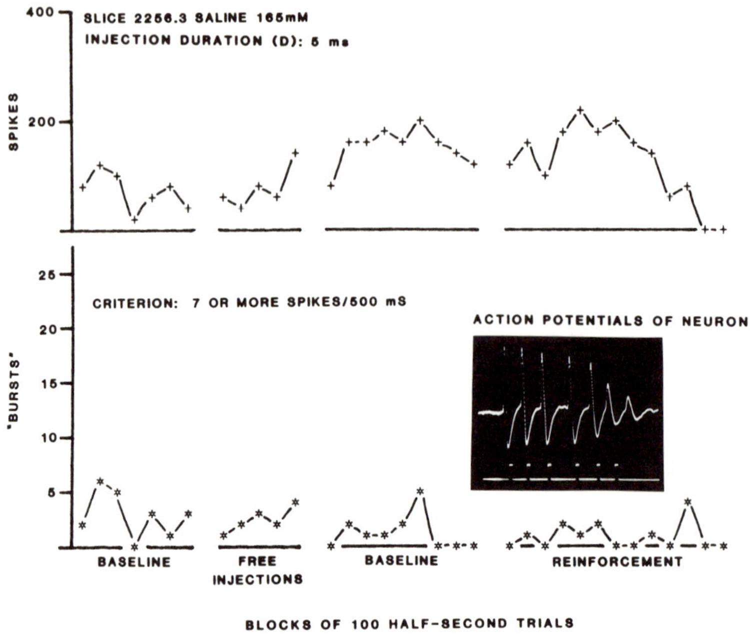

Figure 9.8. Saline control experiment. Failure to obtain evidence of operant conditioning of a pyramidal neuron in dorsal hippocampal slice using local injections of saline as reinforcement. For details, see text and Figure 9.5.

CONCLUSIONS

Cellular applications of dopamine or cocaine to spontaneously active pyramidal cells in slices of rat hippocampus had opposite effects on subsequent firing rates, depending on the activity pattern of the neuron at the time of administration. If the neuron had been firing rapidly just before the injection, the firing rate was increased; if the neuron had been firing slowly or was silent just before the injection, the firing rate was unaffected or decreased. In other words, the action of locally applied dopamine or cocaine on hippocampal cells was activity-related in a way that formally resembles the action of conventional reinforcers on behavior. A food pellet delivered after a lever-press response increases lever pressing, whereas the same pellet delivered independently of the behavior has no effect or even may suppress lever pressing. These observations, therefore, are consistent with the possibility that individual neurons may be operantly conditioned by direct cellular applications of reinforcing transmitters or drugs. If so, the individual neuron may be the functional unit for

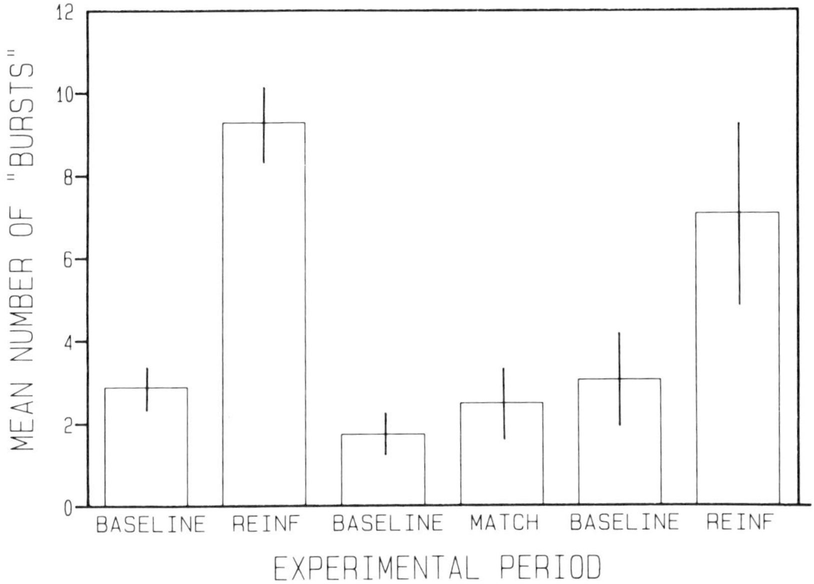

Figure 9.9. Summary of positive dopamine experiments.

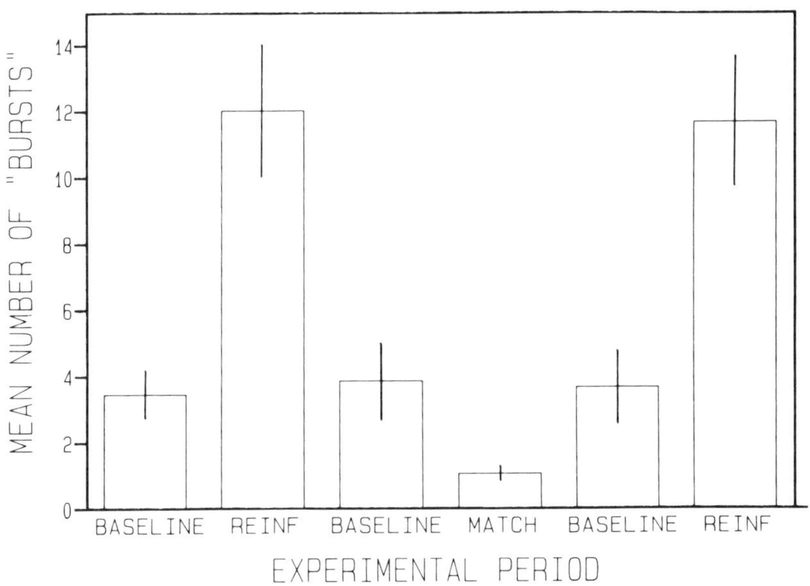

Figure 9.10. Summary of positive cocaine experiments.

Table 9.1
Summary of Hippocampal Slice Experiments

Drug	Dose (mM)	No. of Exps.	Results +	Results ?	Results –
Cocaine	1	48	11	12	25
Cocaine (Free)	1	13	0	0	13
Dopamine	1	17	9	2	6
Dopamine (Free)	1	12	0	1	11
Norepinephrine	1	4	1	1	2
Acetylcholine	1	6	1	1	4
Serotonin	1	3	0	0	3
GABA	1	4	0	0	4
Amphetamine	1	3	0	2	1
Imipramine	1	2	0	0	2
Ethamol	1	3	0	0	3
Saline	165	5	0	0	5

Columns are defined as follows:

+ = conditioning-like changes (increased probability of bursts following reinforcement) plus noncontingent controls,

? = conditioning-like changes but no controls,

– = no evidence of conditioning.

positive reinforcement in the brain, since it is unlikely that a brain cell would display a gratuitous capacity for operant conditioning.

There is already an indication of dopaminergic specificity: included among substances that were ineffective are GABA, serotonin, acetylcholine, imipramine, ethanol, and saline, while cocaine, the only effective reinforcer other than dopamine, is thought to act by enhancing the actions of endogenous dopamine. On a preliminary basis, dopamine seemed to be a more effective agent than norepinephrine. Some evidence suggests that reinforcement schedules may have a different effect in single neurons than they do in the whole animal. Even a simple fixed-ratio 2 schedule caused decrements, rather than increments, in firing rates. Our neuronal preparation also

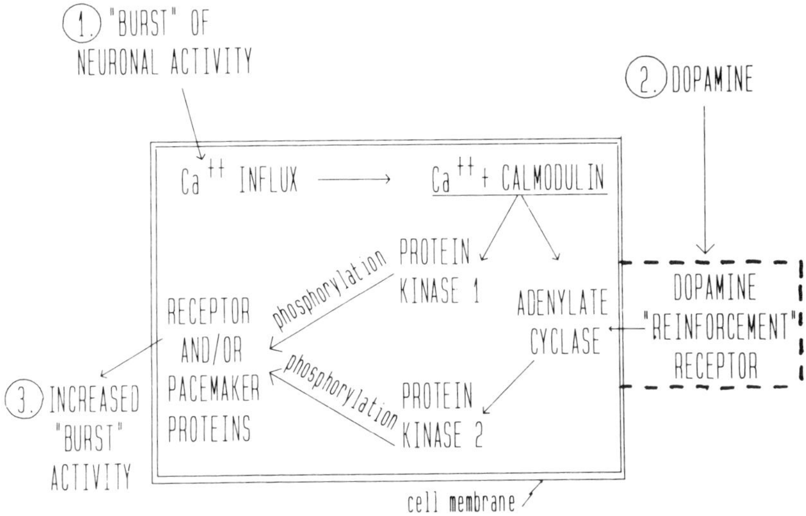

Figure 9.11. Proposed biochemical cascade in neuronal reinforcement.

seemed to differ from conventional operant conditioning with regard to reacquisition after a period of extinction. More rapid reacquisition or "savings," typically observed in behavioral experiments, is not observed in the neuronal studies. The effects of reinforcement schedules and reacquisition thus may reflect properties of neuronal systems rather than of individual cells.

A troublesome feature of these experiments was the fact that relatively high concentrations (1 mM) of dopamine and cocaine were required for reinforcement. However, it should be clear that total drug dose is determined not only by the concentration of the solution injected but also by other injection parameters, such as duration and volume. Because drug injections in our experiment had to be delivered to individual cells in close contingency to bursts of activity, it was necessary to use exceedingly short injection durations (5-20 ms) and small volumes (0.5-3 picoliters). After diffusion to action sites, these minute droplets of drug presumably are diluted to the same concentrations effective in other studies, where lower initial concentrations of drug are applied in greater volumes and for much longer durations.

We have begun to consider the biochemical events that may be involved in cellular reinforcement. What is required is a mechanism that will satisfy the following conditions: 1) if a cell fires, and 2) if the cell's (dopaminergic) reinforcement receptors are then activated, then and only then, 3) will the cellular proteins that control firing be modified (most likely, by phosphorylation) so that the probability of future firing will be increased. Clearly, only recently active cells can be eligible for reinforcement. We do not know which aspect of the activity pattern renders a cell eligible for reinforcement. Four possible markers of recent activity are: depolarization-induced changes in membrane associated proteins, K^+ efflux, Na^+ influx, and Ca^{++} influx. As a working hypothesis, we propose that the influx of Ca^{++} with each "burst" may signal eligibility for reinforcement (Fig. 9.11). Evidence consistent with this hypothesis includes the following: 1) hippocampal pyramidal cells exhibit a remarkable Ca^{++} influx, 10-fold greater than any other cell studied (Krnjevic, 1983), 2) this high-rate Ca^{++} influx may be specifically associated with pyramidal cell bursting activity – the "burst" must contain 3 or more spikes to be effective (Krnjevic, 1983). It has been shown in CA3 cells that the first two spikes are tetrodotoxin sensitive, and presumably mainly mediated by sodium; the third and subsequent spikes are presumably mainly mediated by Ca^{++} (Wong and Prince, 1978), and 3) activation of the large Ca^{++} current by stimulation of CAl inputs has an abrupt threshold, both for stimulation frequency and intensity; such abrupt thresholds are consistent with discrete states of reinforcement eligibility and noneligibility (Krnjevic, 1983). We further assume that the Ca^{++} binds to calmodulin and that the Ca^{++}-calmodulin complex interacts with dopamine-sensitive adenylate cyclase in the cell body so that the cyclase subsequently produces more cAMP in response to dopamine (Greengard, 1978). The final step involving phosphorylation of receptor or pacemaker proteins may be jointly catalyzed by both cAMP-dependent and calcium-calmodulin-dependent protein kinases. Precisely such joint activation of a neuron-specific protein, Protein I, has been reported by Huttner, DeGennaro and Greengard (1981). A similar requirement for activation of receptor or pacemaker proteins that control firing would provide the necessary specificity for reinforcement-induced protein phosphorylation.

In summary, by positing a contingency requirement at two points in the biochemical cascade, the proposed mechanism provides two-fold insurance that only recently active cells can be reinforced. First, because Ca^{++} is required for activation of adenylate cyclase, it insures that only recently active cells will generate high intracellular levels of cAMP in response to dopamine. And secondly, by requiring the joint action of calcium-calmodulin-dependent and cAMP-dependent protein kinases for reinforcement-induced modification of the receptor and pacemaker proteins that control firing, it again insures that Ca++ influx and dopamine receptor stimulation must be contingent.

REFERENCES

Dingledine, R., Dodd, J., and Kelly, J.S. (1980). The *in vitro* brain slice as a useful neurophysiological preparation for intracellular recording. *Journal of Neuroscience Methods*, 2: 323-362.

Feltz, E.E. (1969). Operant conditioning of cortical unit activity. *Science*, 163: 955-958.

Greengard, P. (1978). *Cyclic Nucleotides, Phosphorylated Proteins, and Neuronal Function*, New York: Raven Press.

Hebb, D.O. (1949). *The Organization of Behavior*. New York: John Wiley.

Huttner, W.B., DeGennaro, L. J. and Greengard, P. (1981). Differential phosphorylation of multiple sites in purified protein 1 by cyclic AMP-dependent and calcium-dependent protein kinases. *Journal of Biological Chemistry*, 256: 1482-1488.

Klopf, A.H. (1982). *The Hedonistic Neuron*. Washington, D.C.: Hemisphere Press.

Krnjevic, K. (1983). Personal communication, Gordon Conference.

Olds, J. (1965). Operant conditioning of single unit responses. *Excerpta Medica International Congress Series No. 87*, 372-380.

Schwartzkroin, P.A. (1981). To slice or not to slice. In Kerkut, G. A., and Wheal, H. V. (Eds.), *Electrophysiology of Isolated Mammalian CNS Preparations*. New York: Academic.

Skinner, B.F. (1953). *Science and Human Behavior*. New York: The Free Press.

Stein, L. (1978). Reward transmitters: catecholamines and opioid peptides. In M. A. Lipton, A. DiMascio, and K. F. Killam (Eds.), *Psychopharmacology: A Generation of Progress* (pp. 569-581). New York: Raven Press.

Stein, L., and Belluzzi, J.D. (1979). Brain endorphins: Possible mediators of pleasurable states. In E. Usdin, W.E. Bunney, and N.S. Kline (Eds.), *Endorphins in Mental Health Research.* (pp. 375-389). London: MacMillan Press.

Tyler, T.J. (1980). Brain slice preparation: Hippocampus. *Brain Research Bulletin,* 5: 391-403.

Wong, R.K.S., and Prince, D.A. (1978). Participation of calcium spikes during intrinsic burst firing in hoppocampal neurons. *Brain Research,* 159: 385-390.

Wyler, A.R., and Robbins, C.A. (1980). Operant control of precentral neurons: The role of audio and visual feedback. *Experimental Neurology,* 70: 200-203.

10

The Role of Brain Opioid Systems in Perception of Reward and Anhedonia

TIMOTHY J. COLLIER

In 1954 Olds and Milner (1954) reported that laboratory rats implanted with electrodes in certain brain areas, but not others, would repeatedly press a lever to deliver low-level electrical stimulation to their own brains. This intracranial self-stimulation (ICSS) phenomenon is believed to reflect activation of systems of neurons in the brain that mediate the experience of pleasurable or rewarding properties of environmental stimuli, ranging from the sight of a loved one, to the taste of a favorite food, to the euphoria produced by drugs of abuse.

Over the last several years, ICSS has been used as an experimental tool to study the brain substrates of reward. Initial investigations mapped the brain for the groups of neurons and interconnections that carry the reward message (German and Bowden, 1974; Clavier and Routtenberg, 1980). More recently, efforts have shifted to determining which neurochemical messengers are involved in transmitting reward information along these brain pathways (Wise, 1978; Stein and Beluzzi, 1978; Wise and Bozarth, 1981). The discovery that the brain contains a number of substances that resemble the opiate morphine (Hughes, Smith et al., 1975; Goldstein, 1976; Li and Chung, 1976; Beaumont and Hughes, 1979), both in structure and function, has fueled speculation that neurons

* The author thanks Dr. Aryeh Routtenberg for support, training and collaboration; J. Miller, L. Cahill and D. Barnes for expert technical assistance; J. Goodberlet and P. Weilert for assistance in preparation of the manuscript; and Dr. R. Watson and Mac for graphic design. Research supported by T32-MH 16097 and T32-AG 00107.

containing these endogenous opioid peptides may be involved in perception of pleasure and euphoria. The evidence surrounding this hypothesis will be reviewed, and some speculations will be advanced concerning the role brain opioid system dysfunction could play in the anhedonia of depression.

OPIOIDS AND REWARD

Several lines of evidence support the contention that opioid-containing neurons participate in the transmission of reward information.

Opioid-containing Neurons are Distributed Along Brain Reward Pathways.

As mentioned earlier, a limited number of brain regions support ICSS and are believed to constitute brain circuitry involved in perception of reward. Reconstruction of these rewarding sites indicates that two major brain systems can account for the majority of evidence derived from ICSS mapping studies: a system of neuronal fibers traveling in the medial forebrain bundle of the lateral hypothalamus, and a neural system originating in the dopamine-containing cells of the ventral midbrain tegmentum (Wise, 1980; Shizgal, Bielajew et al., 1980; Wise and Bozarth, 1981). The cells of origin of the medial forebrain bundle system remain unknown, but the direction of transmission appears to be from the forebrain back into the vicinity of the dopamine-containing neurons of the ventral midbrain (Corbett and Wise, 1980). The dopamine-containing system, in general, projects toward the forebrain, sending fibers to a variety of limbic, cortical and basal ganglia structures (Lindvall and Bjorklund, 1974).

Anatomical studies, utilizing the technique of immunocytochemistry, have mapped the distribution of neurons that contain the major opioid peptides: B-endorphin (Bloom, Battenberg, et al., 1978; Watson, Akil et al., 1978), dynorphin (Khachaturian, Watson et al., 1982) and the enkephalins (Khachaturian, Lewis et al., 1983; Uhl, Goodman et al., 1979; Wamsley, Young et al., 1980). Comparison of the distribution of opioid-containing neurons to the map of brain sites supporting reward effects reveals that these neurons parallel the distribution of reward sites. Furthermore, using the map of opioid-containing neurons as a guide for placement of stimulating electrodes for ICSS has led to the identification of previously undetected reward sites (Stein and Beluzzi, 1978). Thus, anatomical studies indicate that opioid-containing neurons and their processes are in a position to be involved in brain reward function.

Opiates Enhance Brain Stimulation Reward.

Initial study of the effects of systemic administration of the opiate drug morphine on responding for rewarding stimulation of the medial forebrain bundle suggested that morphine suppressed reward-related behavior (Olds and Travis, 1960). Subsequent studies revealed that this apparently paradoxical effect was related to a biphasic influence of morphine (Adams, Lorens et al., 1972). The initial suppression of responding for rewarding brain stimulation was related to a sedative action of the opiate lasting for 1-2 hours after injection. If testing continued, a delayed enhancement of reward-related behavior was observed. Furthermore, with repeated daily injections of morphine, tolerance developed to the response-suppressing action of the drug, revealing pure enhancement of responding (Adams, Lorens et al., 1972; Esposito and Kornetsky, 1977). Other studies demonstrated that morphine not only increased the rate of responding for rewarding brain stimulation, but actually decreased the threshold at which responding for rewarding stimulation of the medial forebrain bundle, periaqueductal gray, or ventral midbrain tegmentum occurred (Esposito and Kornetsky, 1977; Esposito, McLean et al., 1979; Kornetsky and Bain, 1982). In addition, this threshold-lowering effect of opiates can be demonstrated even during the initial phase of response suppression which follows acute opiate injection (Gerber, Bozarth et al., 1981). This decreased threshold for obtaining brain stimulation reward is believed to reflect the ability of opiates to enhance activation of brain reward pathways.

The brain site at which morphine has its reward-enhancing effect has been suggested by intracranial microinjection studies. Bilateral injections of morphine or the synthetic enkephalin analogue D-Ala^{2}-Met^{5}-enkephalinamide into the vicinity of the dopamine-containing neurons of the ventral midbrain tegmentum has been shown to yield short latency enhancement of responding for rewarding stimulation of the medial forebrain bundle (Broekkamp, Phillips et al., 1979). Thus, the dopamine neurons of the ventral tegmental area, a brain region previously implicated as the source of one of the major brain reward systems, appears to be one site of action of the opiates' reward-enhancing effect.

Experimental Animals Will Work to Self-administer Opioid Peptides. One of the most compelling findings supporting a role for endogenous opioid peptides in brain mechanisms of reward was the demonstration that rats would press a lever to inject synthetic analogues of the naturally occurring opioid peptides (leucine- and methionine-enkephalin) into the cerebral ventricles of their own brains (Beluzzi and Stein, 1977; Smith, Brown et al., 1982). This behavioral analogue of the brain stimulation reward phenomenon clearly suggested that endogenous opioid peptides had an action in the brain that was pleasurable or rewarding.

Subsequent studies have sought to determine the specific brain areas mediating the rewarding effects of intracranial opioid injections. Two sites previously implicated in the brain stimulation reward phenomenon were found to be sites effective in maintaining opioid self-administration behavior: the lateral hypothalamus in the region of the medial forebrain bundle (Olds and Williams, 1980) and the dopaminergic neurons of the ventral midbrain (Bozarth and Wise, 1981a). An accumulation of evidence suggests that opioid injection into the lateral hypothalamic site may actually act at a distance from this area; possibly at the ventral midbrain tegmentum. When small opioid injections are used, in volumes unlikely to diffuse from the site of injection, experimental animals no longer self-administer opioids into the hypothalamic site, but continue to respond for injections into the dopaminergic ventral midbrain site (Bozarth and Wise, 1980). Furthermore, destruction of neurons in the lateral hypothalamus does not alter self-administration of opiates at this site, suggesting that the rewarding effect of the drug is mediated by some other neuronal population (Britt and Wise, 1981). Thus, evidence to date suggests that the site of rewarding action of self-administered opioids is the dopaminergic cells of the ventral midbrain.

NALOXONE

Up to this point we have discussed evidence regarding opioid effects on reward- related behavior. A necessary complement to these findings is work involving administration of the opiate-receptor blocking agent naloxone. If opioids influence reward-related behavior via an opioid-specific mechanism, the behavior should be modified by opiate receptor blockade. This issue has created controversy, particularly in the interpretation of brain stimulation reward effects. If ICSS behavior derived from sites containing opioid neurons is related to electrically-induced release of endogenous opioids, then naloxone should diminish responding for the rewarding stimulus. Mixed results have been reported. While some authors report consistent decreases in the rate of responding for rewarding brain stimulation following systemic administration of naloxone, particularly from periaqueductal gray sites (Stein and Beluzzi, 1978; Beluzzi and Stein, 1977; Stapleton, Merriman et al., 1979), an equal body of evidence suggests that naloxone has no consistent effect on brain stimulation reward behavior (Stilwell, Levitt et al., 1980; VanDerKooy, LePiane et al., 1977). In addition, studies examining threshold measures for brain stimulation reward also report no effect of naloxone (Kornetsky and Bain, 1982; Esposito, Perry et al., 1980). In contrast to these predominantly null findings on presumed stimulation-induced release of *endogenous* opioids, there is consistent evidence that naloxone blocks or reverses the enhancement of brain stimulation reward produced by systemic administration of *exogenous* opiates (Wise and Bozarth, 1981; Wise, 1980; Kornetsky and Bain, 1982; Esposito, Perry et al., 1980). This combination of results is consistent with the view that the interaction of endogenous opioids with their receptors may not participate *directly* in the expression of reward, but rather, may *modulate* the activity of some other system that actually carries the reward message. Thus, blockade of opiate receptors would not prevent the transmission of rewarding information, but would blunt the enhancement of reward normally produced by activation of opioid systems.

IS OPIOID REWARD REALLY DOPAMINE REWARD?

While the evidence reviewed suggests that opioid-containing neurons participate in brain mechanisms of reward and pleasure, there is little compelling evidence that endogenous opioids are a *necessary* element for expression of reward. Indeed, the majority of the evidence suggests a contrary view: opioids modulate a reward substrate that is dopaminergic (Wise and Bozarth, 1981; Wise, 1980; Wise and Bozarth, 1982). Although circumstantial in nature, several findings support this view.

1. As mentioned earlier, the majority of sites yielding brain stimulation reward behavior fall along the projections of the dopamine neurons of the ventral midbrain tegmentum. Dopamine receptor blockade prevents responding for electrical stimulation of these areas (Wise, 1978) as well as blocking the

rewarding quality of natural rewards like food (Wise, Spindler et al., 1978). Thus, the dopamine system appears to be a *necessary* link in the brain circuitry mediating at least some kinds of reward.

2. While opioid neurons and processes occupy anatomical positions parallel to the dopamine system, they appear to represent a system that may influence dopamine neuron function rather than acting independently. For example, opiate receptors are present on dopamine neurons of the ventral midbrain (Pollard, Llorens et al., 1977; Llorens-Cortes, Pollard et al., 1979), providing a physical substrate for possible opioid modulation of dopamine neuron activity.

3. The site of rewarding action of intracerebrally self-administered opioids appears to be in the vicinity of the dopaminergic cells of the ventral midbrain (Bozarth and Wise, 1981b).

4. With the possible exception of the periaqueductal gray, opiate receptor blockade with naloxone does not appear to diminish brain stimulation reward (Kornetsky and Bain, 1982; Stilwell, Levitt et al., 1980; VanDerKooy, LePiane et al., 1977; Esposito, Perry et al., 1980), but does prevent enhancement of reward behavior by exogenous opiates (Wise and Bozarth, 1981; Wise, 1980; Kornetsky and Bain, 1982; Esposito, Perry et al., 1980). Thus, blockade of endogenous opioids does not preclude expression of reward.

5. The rewarding effects of opiate administration can be blocked by pretreatment with dopamine receptor blockers (Bozarth and Wise, 1981b).

Taken together, this evidence suggests that opioid neurons participate in the neural substrates of reward by direct activation of a dopaminergic link in the reward system (Wise and Bozarth, 1981; Wise, 1980; Wise and Bozarth, 1982), and do not subserve an independent opioid reward-related function.

HIPPOCAMPAL GRANULE CELLS: A DOPAMINE-INDEPENDENT OPIOID REWARD SYSTEM?

The precise role of opioid peptide-containing brain cells in the neural substrates of reward and pleasure remains controversial. Some authors postulate a separable opioid brain reward system (Stein and Beluzzi, 1978), while others suggest that opioid neurons play a minor role, if any, in the mediation of reward-related behavior (VanDerKooy, LePiane et al., 1977).

One obstacle in distinguishing between these possibilities has been the study of brain regions in which opioid elements are in close proximity to portions of the medial forebrain bundle or dopamine system; both of which are implicated in brain reward (Wise, 1978). Study of these areas with ICSS techniques is complicated by the likely coactivation of opioid neurons and elements of these known reward systems.

In an attempt to separate the roles of opioid and dopamine neurons in appreciation of reward, we have studied whether experimental animals will self-administer low-level electrical stimulation to the dentate gyrus granule cells of the dorsal hippocampal formation (Collier and Routtenberg, 1984a). This brain location presents several advantages for study of this problem. First, recent immunohistochemical evidence identifies the granule cells and their mossy fiber axons as regions of dense staining for opioid peptides (Khachaturian, Watson et al., 1982; Khachaturian, Lewis et al., 1983; Gall, Brecha et al., 1981; McGinty, Henricksen et al., 1983). Second, the well-defined anatomy and electrophysiology of this region allows precise placement of stimulating electrodes into the granule cell layer, ensuring relatively selective stimulation of these opioid-containing neurons. Third, the direct participation of dopamine neurons in reward-related behavior derived from granule cell stimulation is unlikely: Dopamine is not anatomically detectable in this region (Lindvall and Bjorklund, 1974). Thus, careful use of low electric currents applied through electrodes positioned precisely in the granule cell layer should allow examination of reward behavior derived from preferential activation of the endogenous opioid system in this area.

A single monopolar electrode (78.7 μM diameter nichrome wire) was electrophysiologically guided, as described previously (Collier, Miller et al., 1982), into the granule cell layer of the dorsal dentate gyrus of male albino rats. All 17 electrodes analyzed in this study were histologically confirmed to be located in the granule cell layer (11 in the dorsal limb, 6 in the ventral limb).

Subjects were tested in an operant chamber in which depression of a lever delivered a 500 msec duration train of 60 Hz sine wave electrical stimulation at 10 μA peak amplitude. Animals were exposed to the test situation on three overnight sessions, and thereafter had access to brain stimulation during one daily 15-minute duration session.

Reward-related behavior also was studied during systemic challenge by the opiate antagonist naloxone. Naloxone-HCl (Endo Labs; 0.01, 0.05, 0.10, 0.50, 1.00, 2.00, 5.00 mg/kg) was dissolved in 0.9% saline vehicle and administered by intraperitoneal injection 10-15 minutes prior to brain stimulation tests. At least one day of vehicle injection intervened between drug tests. Statistical differences between mean response rates of control animals and drug-treated animals were assessed with a one-way analysis of variance followed by Neuman-Keuls testing to highlight individual differences.

We have found that animals will lever-press to self-administer granule cell stimulation. They exhibit significantly higher mean peak response rates than unoperated control animals (granule cell stimulation: 49.06 $\pm$12.79 responses/15 min.; unoperated controls: 11.80 $\pm$1.07 responses/15 min.; $p < .01$).

Naloxone pretreatment decreased self-administration of granule cell stimulation (Figure 10.1). This is consistent with the presence of opioid immunoreactivity associated with these cells, and supports the view that opioid mechanisms are involved in maintenance of this reward-related behavior. Naloxone reduced responding in a dose-related manner, with a dose of 1.0 mg/kg producing a significant decrease in response rate (-40%), and 5.0 mg/kg producing response levels equivalent to those maintained by animals that are not receiving brain stimulation. It is noteworthy that subjects appeared behaviorally normal in other respects following naloxone treatment. When placed in the test chambers these animals immediately initiated responding, but tended to discontinue lever-pressing after the first 5 minutes of the session. The same doses which significantly depressed responding for granule cell stimulation had no effect on the low response rates emitted by operant controls, nor did these doses affect high rates of responding for medial forebrain bundle stimulation examined in a separate study. Thus, naloxone suppression of granule cell reward behavior does not appear to be attributable to non-specific behavioral depression.

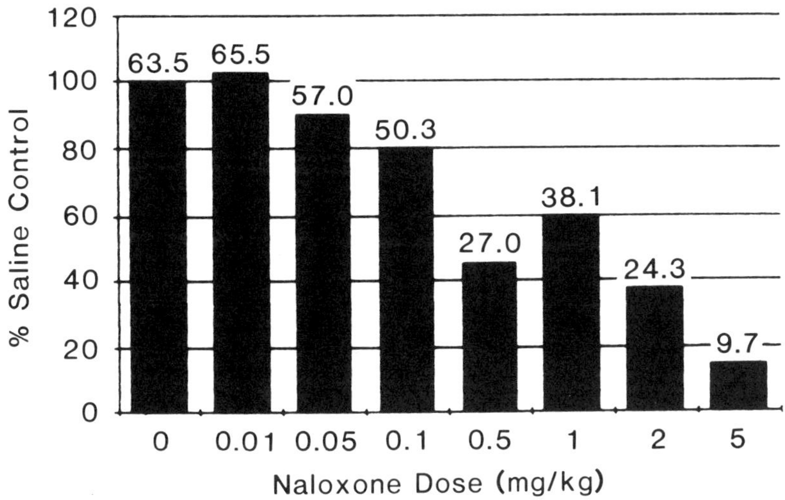

Figure 10.1. Opiate-receptor blockade by systemic treatment with naloxone reduces granule cell self-stimulation in a dose-dependent manner. The histogram depicts the dose-related response supression obtained following naloxone treatment as a percentage of the response rate obtained following pretreatment with the saline vehicle (naloxone dose = 0). Numbers on top of bars are mean number of responses per 15 min. test under each treatment condition. Means are derived from a variable number of tests for each condition: Naloxone dose: 0 = 75 tests, 0.01 = 8 tests, 0.05 = 4 tests, 0.10 = 9 tests, 0.50 = 3 tests, 1.00 = 12 tets, 2.00 = 6 tests, 5.00 = 3 tests.

These results provide one of the clearest indications that an identifiable cell population is part of a system involved in mediation of reward-related behavior. In addition, we suggest that animals lever-pressing for granule cell stimulation are self- administering their own opioid peptides contained in these neurons. If activation of the opioid synapse is prevented by naloxone, reward is not expressed. This is observed at the 5.0 mg/kg dose of naloxone where responding for granule cell stimulation is reduced to levels comparable to rates of control animals receiving no brain stimulation.

It is important to note that unlike other opioid sites studied in relation to reward behavior, the granule cell layer is not penetrated by, or in close proximity to, elements of the dopaminergic and medial forebrain bundle systems believed to mediate reward, and thus these systems could not be directly activated by our stimulation. Furthermore, these opioid neurons constitute a local hippocampal connection and do not project directly (monosynaptically) upon either of these postulated reward systems.

Reward-related neurons in the hippocampal formation may constitute a system in which opioid neurons are a *necessary* link in the neural reward chain. Admittedly, direct evidence supporting this contention is minimal at present. We have demonstrated that opiate receptor blockade prevents reward-related responding for granule cell stimulation. In addition, the direct involvement of dopamine neurons in reward-related behavior derived from hippocampal circuitry is inconsistent with the anatomy of the region. Experimental animals will self-administer electrical stimulation to all portions of the entorhinal cortex (Collier, Kurtzman et al., 1977; Ott, Destrade et al., 1980) perforant path (Collier, Miller et al., 1980)→dentate gyrus (Collier and Routtenberg, 1984a)→CA3 pyramidal cells (Campbell, Milgram et al., 1978; Ursin, Ursin et al., 1966)→CA1 pyramidal cells (Ursin, Ursin et al., 1966) entorhinal cortex circuit. But while there is a dopamine projection to a portion of the lateral entorhinal cortex (Collier and Routtenberg, 1977), the remainder of this circuit contains no anatomically demonstrable dopamine innervation (Lindvall and Bjorklund, 1974). In contrast, opioid peptides are present in neurons and the major fiber pathways throughout the hippocampal circuit: including entorhinal cortex neurons that give rise to the perforant path, the perforant path projection to the dentate gyrus, dentate gyrus granule cells and their mossy fiber projection to the hippocampal CA3 pyramidal cells (Khachaturian, Watson et al., 1982; Khachaturian, Lewis et al., 1983; Gall, Brecha et al., 1981; McGinty, Henricksen et al., 1983). It remains to be determined whether experimental animals will self-inject opioids directly into these hippocampal sites, providing direct evidence in support of a critical opioid substrate for reward behavior derived from this area.

In summary, a convincing body of evidence has accumulated favoring the view that opioids exert their reward-enhancing influence on subcortical reward systems by activation of the dopamine pathway originating in the ventral midbrain tegmentum. In addition, however, the demonstration of naloxone-sensitive reward behavior derived from hippocampal granule cells, coupled with the absence of dopamine in the hippocampal circuit, provides an initial indication that a dopamine-independent opioid reward system may exist in limbic cortex.

OPIOID SYSTEM DYSFUNCTION AND ANHEDONIA: A SPECULATIVE ROLE IN AFFECT DEFICIT STATES

This final section of the chapter will depart from the various arguments concerning the specific role opioid-containing neurons play in brain reward function, and advance some speculations concerning the involvement of opioid system dysfunction in affect deficit states. Whether or not opioid neurons are a necessary element in mediating perception of reward, it is clear that brain reward systems are accessed by opiate drugs, and this access is mediated by opioid receptors in the brain. Accordingly, dysfunction of brain opioid systems may contribute to psychological states in which perception of pleasure and reward are altered. One such altered mental state is depression. Symptoms of depression can include a loss of the ability to feel pleasure. Ideas, activities and relationships that usually bring pleasure can be perceived as empty or hollow (Berger, 1978). In particular, then, evidence relating to possible *decreased* function of opioid systems in affect deficit states will be reviewed. While direct study of opioid system involvement in the anhedonia of human depression is just beginning, some interesting clues can be derived from experimentation on animals.

The first clue relates to an apparent role for opioid peptides in selective attention and reactivity to novel environmental stimuli. Studies mapping the distribution of opiate receptor sites in functionally defined regions of primate cerebral cortex (Lewis, Mishkin et al., 1981) may be of particular relevance to opioid system function in humans. Mu and delta opiate receptors were mapped by studying the specific binding of ^{3}H-naloxone and ^{3}H-enkephalin, respectively, in rhesus monkey cortex. An interesting pattern emerged. Whereas delta receptors (^{3}H-enkephalin binding sites) were distributed evenly throughout the cortex, mu receptors (^{3}H-naloxone binding sites) were sparse in cortical areas devoted to initial registration of sensory events, but increased markedly in cortical regions devoted to processing of increasingly complex information. It is interesting that mu opiate receptors were concentrated in cortical regions of recent evolutionary expansion (Lewis, Mishkin et al., 1981; Wise and Herkenham, 1982), further supporting the view that opiate modulation of cortex may have evolved to participate in brain systems which process complex information. It is known that the cortical areas that are rich in mu receptors encode reward-related aspects of sensory information in primates (Rothblat and Pribram, 1972; Nuwer and

Pribram, 1979), and that opiate administration in humans affects electrophysiological measures of attention (Davis, Buchbaum et al., 1980). Based on this information, the authors propose that increased opioid modulation of association cortex may reflect opioid involvement in the process of selective attention (Lewis, Mishkin et al., 1981). Specifically, opioid neurons may help integrate information regarding reward contingencies and emotional states with sensory stimuli, to aid in the process of choosing stimuli to be attended to.

Research in rodents also is consistent with a role for opioids in modulating responsiveness to the environment. Systemic administration of the opiate-receptor blocker naloxone reduced exploratory and social activity (File, 1980; Katz and Gelbart, 1978; Arnsten and Segal, 1979). Of particular interest was the finding that naloxone reduced responding in a situation where animals could press a lever to induce environmental novelty (change illumination and sound in the experimental chamber) (Katz and Gelbart, 1978). The authors suggest that blockade of opiate receptors interferes with the rewarding properties of environmental stimuli. Although a role for opioids in association of reward or emotional states with sensory information is speculative at present, the blunting of pleasure derived from interactions with peers and the environment that would follow disruption of this function is consistent with the symptoms of affect deficit states.

A second clue relates to the neurochemistry of electroconvulsive therapy (ECT). ECT results in significant improvement of symptoms of certain types of depression (Crow and Johnstone, 1978). While the therapeutic influence of ECT has been linked to enhanced release and utilization of brain norepinephrine (Kety, Javoy et al., 1967; Musacchio, Julou et al., 1969), it is noteworthy that ECT also stimulates release of brain opioids (Green, Peralta et al., 1978; Hong, Gillin et al., 1979; Tortella and Cowan, 1982). Thus, the antidepressant effects of ECT may be mediated in part by stimulation of endogenous opioid neurons.

Brain opioid systems are believed to be involved in a variety of functions besides perception of reward (Olson, Olson et al., 1981). Accordingly, widespread opioid system dysfunction may alter a variety of opioid-related functions and behaviors in addition to effects on reward. For example, it has been suggested that brain opioid systems participate in the process of forgetting (Collier and Routtenberg, 1984b; Izquierdo, Dias et al., 1980) Indeed, previous evidence suggests that neuron systems involved in reward are also involved in memory function (Routtenberg, 1978), and that the hippocampal granule cells, in particular, are involved both in reward-related behavior and in removal of information from memory (Collier and Routtenberg, 1984a; Collier and Routtenberg, 1984b). It is intriguing to envision the consequences of opioid system dysfunction where the dysfunction involves this cell population. Potentially, perception of reward would be diminished in combination with impairment of the ability to forget. In this psychological state, not only would little pleasure be derived from daily events and interactions, but these negative experiences would linger in memory, extending the subjective time-course of the potentially depressing episode.

Finally, it is important to recall that disorders involving affect deficit states are complex and variable in their symptomatology. It is almost certain that their etiology involves imbalances in more than one neurochemical system, and that the systems involved may vary between individuals. In the case of depression, disruption of brain norepinephrine (Bunney and Davis, 1965; Schildkraut, 1965), serotonin (Lapin and Oxenkrug, 1969), acetylcholine (Janowsky, el-Yousef et al., 1972) and dopamine (Bunney, VanKammen et al., 1979) systems all have been proposed. The addition of brain opioid systems to this list does nothing to simplify the issue, but may ultimately prove useful in developing therapies for certain types of affect deficit states.

REFERENCES

Adams, W.J., Lorens, S.A. and Mitchell, C.L. (1972). Morphine enhances lateral hypothalamic self-stimulation in the rat. *Proc. Soc. Exper. Biol. Med.*, 140:770-771.

Arnsten, A.T. and Segal, D.S. (1979). Naloxone alters locomotion and interactions with environmental stimuli. *Life Sci.*, 25:1035-1042.

Beaumont, A. and Hughes, J. (1979). Biology of opioids and peptides. *Ann. Rev. Pharmacol. Toxicol.*, 19:245-267.

Beluzzi, J.D. and Stein, L. (1977). Enkephalin may mediate euphoria and drive-reduction reward. *Nature*, 266:556-558.

Berger, P.A. (1978). Medical treatment of mental illness. *Science*, 200:974-981.

Bloom, F.E., Battenberg, E., Rossier, J., Ling, N. and Guillemin, R. (1978). Neurons containing beta-endorphin in rat brain exist separately from those containing enkephalin: Immunocytochemical studies. *Proc. Natl. Acad. Sci.*, (U.S.A.), 75:1591-1595.

Bozarth, M.A. and Wise, R.A. (1980). Intracranial self-administration of morphine into various brain regions in rats. *Soc. Neurosci.*, 6:309.

Bozarth, M.A. and Wise, R.A. (1981a). Intracranial self-administration of morphine into the ventral tegmental area in rats. *Life Sci.*, 28:551-555.

Bozarth, M.A. and Wise, R.A. (1981b). Heroin reward is dependent on a dopaminergic substrate. *Life Sci.*, 29:1881-1886.

Britt, M.D. and Wise, R.A. (1981). Opiate rewarding action: Independence of the cells of the lateral hypothalamus. *Brain Res.*, 222:213-217.

Broekkamp, C.L., Phillips, A.G. and Cools, A.R. (1979). Facilitation of self-stimulation behavior following intracerebral microinjections of opiods into the ventral tegmental area. *Pharmacol. Biochem. Behav.*, 11:289-295.

Bunney, W.E., Jr. and Davis, J.M. (1965). Norepinephrine in depressive reactions. A review. *Arch. Gen. Psychiat.*, 13:483-494.

Bunney, W.E., VanKammen, D.P., Post, R.M. and Garland, B.L. (1979). A possible role for dopamine in schizophrenic and manic-depressive illness. A review of evidence. In E. Usdin, I.J. Kopin and J. Barchas (Eds.), *Catecholamines: Basic and Clinical Frontiers II.* Elmsford, N.Y.: Pergamon Press, pp. 1807-1819.

Campbell, K.A., Milgram, N.W. and Christoff, J.K. (1978). Plasticity in the reinforcing consequences of hippocampal stimulation. *Brain Res.*, 159:458-462.

Clavier, R.M. and Routtenberg, A. (1980). In search of reinforcement pathways: A neuroanatomical odyssey. In A. Routtenberg (Ed.), *Biology of Reinforcement: Facets of Brain Stimulation Reward.* New York: Academic Press, pp. 81-107.

Collier, T.J., Kurtzman, S. and Routtenberg, A. (1977). Intracranial self-stimulation derived from entorhinal cortex. *Brain Res.*, 137:188-196.

Collier, T.J., Miller, J.S. and Routtenberg, A. (1980). Electrophysiological guidance of hippocampal electrodes for intracranial self-stimulation "I.C.S.S." in angular bundle, perforant path, and dentate gyrus. *Soc. Neurosci.*, 6:110.

Collier, T.J., Miller, J.S., Travis, J. and Routtenberg, A. (1982). Dentate gyrus granule cells and memory: Electrical stimulation disrupts memory for places of reward. *Behav. Neural Biol.*, 34:227-239.

Collier, T.J. and Routtenberg, A. (1977). Entorhinal cortex: Catecholamine fluorescence and Nissl staining of Vibratome sections. *Brain Res.*, 128:354-360.

Collier, T.J. and Routtenberg, A. (1984a). Selective impairment of declarative memory following stimulation of dentate gyrus granule cells: A naloxone-sensitive effect. *Brain Res.*, 310:384-387.

Collier, T.J. and Routtenberg, A. (1984b). Electrical self-stimulation of dentate gyrus granule cells. *Behav. Neural. Biol.*, 42:85-90.

Corbett, D. and Wise, R.A. (1980). Intracranial self-stimulation in relation to the ascending noradrenergic fiber systems of the pontine tegmentum and caudal midbrain: A moveable electrode mapping study. *Brain Res.*, 185:1-15.

Crow, T.J. and Johnstone, E.C. (1978). ECT - does it work? *Trends Neurosci.*, 1:51-53.

Davis, G.C., Buchbaum, M.S. and Bunney, W.E., Jr. (1980). Alterations of evoked potentials link research in attention dysfunction to peptide response symptoms of schizophrenia. *Adv. Biochem. Psychopharmacol.*, 22:473-487.

Esposito, R. and Kornetsky, C. (1977). Morphine lowering of self-stimulation thresholds: Lack of tolerance with long-term administration. *Science*, 195:189-191.

Esposito, R.U., McLean, S. and Kornetsky, C. (1979). Effects of morphine on intracranial self-stimulation to various brain stem loci. *Brain Res.*, 168:425-429.

Esposito, R.U., Perry, W. and Kornetsky, C. (1980). Effects of d-amphetamine and naloxone on brain stimulation reward. *Psychopharmacol.*, 69:187-191.

File, S.E. (1980). Naloxone reduces social and exploratory activity in the rat. *Psycho pharmacol.*, 71:41-44.

Gall, C., Brecha, N., Karten, H.J. and Chang, K-J. (1981). Localization of enkephalin-like immunoreactivity to identified axonal and neuronal populations of the rat hippocampus. *J. Comp. Neurol.*, 198:335-350.

Gerber, G.J., Bozarth, M.A. and Wise, R.A. (1981). Small dose intravenous heroin facilitates hypothalamic self-stimulation without response suppression in rats. *Life Sci.*, 28:557-562.

German, D.C. and Bowden, D.M. (1974). Catecholamine systems as the neural substrate for intracranial self stimulation: A hypothesis. *Brain Res.*, 73:381-419.

Goldstein, A. (1976). Opioid peptides (endorphins) in pituitary and brain. *Science*, 193:1081-1086.

Green, A.R., Peralta, E., Hong, J.S., Mao, C.C., Atterwill, C.K. and Costa, E. (1978). Alterations in GABA metabolism and Met-enkephalin content in rat brain following repeated electroconvulsive shocks. *J. Neurochem.*, 31:607-611.

Hong, J.S., Gillin, J.C., Yang, H-Y.T. and Costa, E. (1979). Repeated electroconvulsive shocks and the brain content of endorphins. *Brain Res.*, 177:273-278.

Hughes, J., Smith, T.W., Kosterlitz, H., Fothergill, L.A., Morgan, B.A. and Morris, H.R. (1975). Identification of two pentapeptides from the brain with potent opiate agonist activity. *Nature*, 258:577-579.

Izquierdo, I., Dias, R.D., Souza, D.O., Carrasco, M.A., Elizabetsky, E. and Perry, M.L.(1980). The role of opioid peptides in memory and learning. *Behav. Brain Res.*, 1:451-468.

Janowsky, D.S., el-Yousef, M.K., Davis, J.M. and Sekerke, H.J. (1972). A cholinergic- adrenergic hypothesis of mania and depression. *Lancet*, 2:632-635.

Katz, R.J. and Gelbart, J. (1978). Endogenous opiates and behavioral responses to environmental novelty. *Behav. Biol.*, 24:41-44.

Kety, S.S., Javoy, F., Thierry, A.M., Julou, L. and Glowinski, J. (1967). A sustained effect of electroconvulsive shock on the turnover of norepinephrine in the central nervous system of the rat. *Proc. Natl. Acad. Sci.* (U.S.A.), 58:1249-1254.

Khachaturian, H., Lewis, M.E., Hollt, V. and Watson, S.J. (1983). Telencephalic enkephalinergic systems in the rat brain. *J. Neurosci.*, 3:844-855.

Khachaturian, H., Watson, S.J., Lewis, M.E., Coy, D., Goldstein, A. and Akil, H. (1982). Dynorphin immunocytochemistry in the rat central nervous system. *Peptides*, 3:941-954.

Kornetsky, C. and Bain, G. (1982). Biobehavioral bases of the reinforcing properties of opiate drugs. *Annals N.Y. Acad. Sci.*, 398:241-259.

Lapin, I.P. and Oxenkrug, G.F. (1969). Intensification of the central serotoninergic processes as a possible determinant of the thymoleptic effect. *Lancet*, 1:132-136.

Lewis, M.E., Mishkin, M., Bragin, E., Brown, R.M., Pert, C.B., and Pert, A. (1981). Opiate receptor gradients in monkey cerebral cortex: Correspondence with sensory processing hierarchies. *Science*, 211:1166-1169.

Li, C.H. and Chung, D. (1976). Isolation and structure of an untriakontapeptide with opiate activity from camel pituitary glands. *Proc. Natl. Acad. Sci.* (U.S.), 73:1145-1148

Lindvall, O. and Bjorklund, A. (1974). The organization of the ascending catecholamine neuron systems in the rat brain as revealed by the glyoxylic acid fluorescence method. *Acta Physiol. Scand.*, Suppl. 412:1-48.

Llorens-Cortes, C., Pollard, H. and Schwartz, J.C. (1979). Localization of opiate receptors in substantia nigra evidence by lesion studies. *Neurosci. Lett.*, 12:165-170.

McGinty, J.F., Henricksen, S.J., Goldstein, A., Terenius, L. and Bloom, F.E. (1983). Dynorphin is contained within hippocampal mossy fibers: Immunochemical alterations after kainic acid administration and colchicine-induced neurotoxicity. *Proc. Nat. Acad. Sci.*, 80:589-593.

Musacchio, J.M., Julou, L., Kety, S.S. and Glowinski, J. (1969). Increase in rat brain tyrosine hydroxylase activity produced by electroconvulsive shock. *Proc. Natl. Acad. Sci.* (U.S.A.), 63:1117-1119.

Nuwer, M.R. and Pribram, K.H. (1979). Role of the inferotemporal cortex in visual selective attention. *EEG Clin. Neurophysiol.*, 46:389-400.

Olds, J. Milner, P. (1954): Positive reinforcement produced by electrical stimulation of septal area and other regions of rat brain. *J. Comp. Physiol. Psychol.*, 47:419-427.

Olds, J. and Travis, R.P. (1960). Effects of chlorpromazine, meprobamate, pentobarbital and morphine on self-stimulation. *J. Pharmacol. Exper. Ther.*, 128:397-404.

Olds, M.E. and Williams, K.N. (1980). Self-administration of D-Ala2-Met-enkephalinamide hypothalamic self-stimulation sites. *Brain Res.*, 194:155-170.

Olson, G.A., Olson, R.D., Kastin, A.J. and Coy, D.H. (1981). Endogenous opiates. *Peptides*, 2:349-369.

Ott, T., Destrade, C. and Ruthrich, H. (1980). Induction of self-stimulation behavior derived from a brain region lacking in dopaminergic innervation. *Behav. Neural Biol.*, 28:512-516.

Pollard, H., Llorens, C., Bonnet, J.J., Costentin, J. and Schwartz, J.C. (1977). Opiate receptors on mesolimbic dopaminergic neurons. *Neurosci. Lett.*, 7:295-299.

Rothblat, L. and Pribram, K.H. (1972). Selective attention: Input filter or response selection? An electrophysiological analysis. *Brain Res.*, 39:427-436.

Routtenberg, A. (1978). The reward system of the brain. *Sci. Amer.*, 239:154-164.

Schildkraut, J.J. (1965). The catecholamine hypothesis of affective disorders: A review of supporting evidence. *Amer. J. Psychiat.*, 122:509-522.

Shizgal, P., Bielajew, C., Corbett, D., Skelton, R. and Yeomans, J. (1980). Behavioral methods for inferring anatomical linkage between rewarding brain stimulation sites. *J. Comp. Physiol. Psychol.*, 94:227-237.

Smith, B.R., Brown, Z.W. and Amit, Z. (1982). Intraventricular self-administration of leucine-enkephalin by laboratory rats. *Life Sci.*, 31:1527-1530.

Stapleton, J.M., Merriman, V.J., Coogle, C.L., Gelbard, S.D. and Reid, L.D. (1979). Naloxone reduces pressing for intracranial stimulation of sites in the periaqueductal gray area, accumbens nucleas, substantia nigra, and lateral hypothalamus. *Physiol. Psychol*, 7:427-436.

Stein, L. and Beluzzi (1978). Brain endorphins and the sense of well-being and psychobiological hypothesis. In E. Costa and M. Trabucchi (Eds.), *Advances in Bio chemical Psychopharmacology*, Vol. 18. New York: Raven Press, pp. 299-311.

Stilwell, D.J., Levitt, R.A., Horn, C.A., Irvin, M.D., Gross, K., Parsons, D.S., Scott, R.H. and Bradley, E.L. (1980). Naloxone and shuttlebox self-stimulation in the rat. *Pharmacol. Biochem. Behav.*, 13:739-742.

Tortella, F.C. and Cowan, A. (1982). EEG, EMG and behavioral evidence for the involvement of endorphin systems in postictal events after electroconvulsive shock in rats. *Life Sci.*, 31:881-888.

Uhl, G.R., Goodman, R.R., Kuhar, M.J., Childers, S.R. and Snyder, S.H. (1979). Immunohistochemical mapping of enkephalin containing cell bodies, fibers and nerve terminals in the brain stem of the rat. *Brain Res.*, 166:75-94.

Ursin, R., Ursin, H. and Olds, J. (1966). Self-stimulation of hippocampus in rats. *J. Comp. Physiol. Psychol.*, 61:353-359.

VanKerKooy, D., LePiane, F.G. and Phillips A.G. (1977). Apparent independence of opiate reinforcement and electrical self-stimulation system in rat brain. *Life Sci.*, 20:981-986.

Wamsley, J.K., Young, W.S. III and Kuhar, M.J. (1980). Immunohistochemical localization of enkephalin in rat forebrain. *Brain Res.*, 190:153-174.

Watson, S.J., Akil, H., Richard, C.W. and Barchas, J.D. (1978). Evidence for two separate opiate peptide neuronal systems. *Nature*, 275:226-228.

Wise, R.A. (1978). Catecholamine theories of reward: A critical review. *Brain Res.*, 152:215-247.

Wise, R.A. (1980). Action of drugs of abuse on brain reward systems. *Pharmacol. Biochem. Behav.*, 13:213-223.

Wise, R.A. and Bozarth, M.A. (1981). Brain substrates for reinforcement and drug self-administration. *Prog. Neuro-Psychopharmacol.*, 5:467-474.

Wise, R.A. and Bozarth, M.A. (1982). Action of drugs of abuse on brain reward systems: An update with specific attention to opiates. *Pharmacol. Biochem. Behav.*, 17:239-243.

Wise, R.A., Spindler, J., DeWitt, H. and Gerber, G.J. (1978). Neuroleptic-induced "anhedonia" in rats: Pimozide blocks reward quality of food. *Science*, 201:262-264.

Wise, S.P. and Herkenham, M. (1982). Opiate receptor distribution in the cerebral cortex of Rhesus monkey. *Science*, 218:387-388.

Index